Current Topics in Microbiology and Immunology

Volume 352

Current Topics in Microbiology and Immunology

Previously published volumes

Further volumes can be found at www.springer.com

Vol. 322: **Romeo, Tony (Ed.)**:
Bacterial Biofilms. 2008.
ISBN 978-3-540-75417-6

Vol. 323: **Tracy, Steven; Oberste, M. Steven; Drescher, Kristen M. (Eds.)**:
Group B Coxsackieviruses. 2008.
ISBN 978-3-540-75545-6

Vol. 324: **Nomura, Tatsuji; Watanabe, Takeshi; Habu, Sonoko (Eds.)**:
Humanized Mice. 2008
ISBN 978-3-540-75646-0

Vol. 325: **Shenk, Thomas E.; Stinski, Mark F. (Eds.)**:
Human Cytomegalovirus. 2008.
ISBN 978-3-540-77348-1

Vol. 326: **Reddy, Anireddy S. N.; Golovkin, Maxim (Eds.)**:
Nuclear pre-mRNA processing in plants. 2008
ISBN 978-3-540-76775-6

Vol. 327: **Manchester, Marianne; Steinmetz Nicole F. (Eds.)**:
Viruses and Nanotechnology. 2008.
ISBN 978-3-540-69376-5

Vol. 328: **van Etten, (Ed.)**:
Lesser Known Large dsDNA Viruses. 2008.
ISBN 978-3-540-68617-0

Vol. 329: **Griffin, Diane E.; Oldstone, Michael B. A. (Eds.)**: Measles. 2009
ISBN 978-3-540-70522-2

Vol. 330: **Griffin, Diane E.; Oldstone, Michael B. A. (Eds.)**:
Measles. 2009.
ISBN 978-3-540-70616-8

Vol. 331: **Villiers, E. M. de (Ed.)**:
TT Viruses. 2009. ISBN 978-3-540-70917-8

Vol. 332: **Karasev A. (Ed.)**:
Plant produced Microbial Vaccines. 2009.
ISBN 978-3-540-70857-5

Vol. 333: **Compans, Richard W.; Orenstein, Walter A. (Eds.)**:
Vaccines for Pandemic Influenza. 2009.
ISBN 978-3-540-92164-6

Vol. 334: **McGavern, Dorian; Dustin, Micheal (Eds.)**:
Visualizing Immunity. 2009.
ISBN 978-3-540-93862-0

Vol. 335: **Levine, Beth; Yoshimori, Tamotsu; Deretic, Vojo (Eds.)**:
Autophagy in Infection and Immunity. 2009.
ISBN 978-3-642-00301-1

Vol. 336: **Kielian, Tammy (Ed.)**:
Toll-like Receptors: Roles in Infection and Neuropathology. 2009.
ISBN 978-3-642-00548-0

Vol. 337: **Sasakawa, Chihiro (Ed.)**:
Molecular Mechanisms of Bacterial Infection via the Gut. 2009.
ISBN 978-3-642-01845-9

Vol. 338: **Rothman, Alan L. (Ed.)**:
Dengue Virus. 2009.
ISBN 978-3-642-02214-2

Vol. 339: **Spearman, Paul; Freed, Eric O. (Eds.)**:
HIV Interactions with Host Cell Proteins. 2009.
ISBN 978-3-642-02174-9

Vol. 340: **Saito, Takashi; Batista, Facundo D. (Eds.)**:
Immunological Synapse. 2010.
ISBN 978-3-642-03857-0

Vol. 341: **Bruserud, Øystein (Ed.)**:
The Chemokine System in Clinical and Experimental Hematology. 2010.
ISBN 978-3-642-12638-3

Vol. 342: **Arvin, Ann M. (Ed.)**:
Varicella-zoster Virus. 2010.
ISBN 978-3-642-12727-4

Vol. 343: **Johnson, John E. (Ed.)**:
Cell Entry by Non-Enveloped Viruses. 2010.
ISBN 978-3-642-13331-2

Vol. 345: **Simon, M. Celeste (Ed.)**:
Diverse Effects of Hypoxia on Tumor Progression. 2010.
ISBN 978-3-642-13328-2

Vol. 346: **Christian Rommel; Bart Vanhaesebroeck; Peter K. Vogt (Ed.)**:
Phosphoinositide 3-kinase in Health and Disease. 2010.
ISBN 978-3-642-13662-7

Vol. 347: **Christian Rommel; Bart Vanhaesebroeck; Peter K. Vogt (Ed.)**:
Phosphoinositide 3-kinase in Health and Disease. 2010.
ISBN 978-3-642-14815-6

Vol. 348: **Lyubomir Vassilev; David Fry (Eds.)**:
Small-Molecule Inhibitors of Protein-Protein Interactions. 2011.
ISBN 978-3-642-17082-9

Vol. 349: **Michael Kartin (Eds.)**:
NF-kB in Health and Disease. 2011.
ISBN: 978-3-642-16017-2

Vol. 350: **Rafi Ahmed; Tasuku Honjo (Eds.)**
Negative Co-receptors and Ligands
ISBN: 978-3-642-19545-7

Rudolf Valenta · Robert L. Coffman
Editors

Vaccines against Allergies

Responsible series editor: Fritz Melchers

Springer

Prof. Dr. Rudolf Valenta
Christian Doppler Laboratory
for Allergy Research
Medical University of Vienna
1090 Vienna
Austria
e-mail: Rudolf.valenta@meduniwien.ac.at

Robert L. Coffman Ph.D.
Dynavax Technologies
Seventh Street 2929 Suite 100
Berkeley, CA 94710
USA
e-mail: rcoffman@dynavax.com

ISSN 0070-217X
ISBN 978-3-642-20053-3 e-ISBN 978-3-642-20054-0
DOI 10.1007/978-3-642-20054-0
Springer Heidelberg Dordrecht London New York

Library of Congress Control Number: 2011936232

Cover design: Deblik, Berlin

Printed on acid-free paper

Springer is part of Springer Science+Business Media (www.springer.com)

Preface

Current Strategies for Allergen-Specific Immunotherapy at its Centenary

We are celebrating this year the 100 years' anniversary of allergen-specific immunotherapy. In 1911 Leonard Noon published his seminal work "Prophylactic inoculation against hay fever" describing his attempts to achieve active immunity against "grass pollen toxin" by administering increasing doses of grass pollen extract before the grass pollen season to allergic patients. Although it was unknown at that time that allergy represents an immunological hypersensitivity disease, the treatment was effective and many observations made by Noon remained valid until today. Noon noted side effects and that initially increased sensitivity was followed by tolerance which lasted for approximately one year.

Today allergen-specific immunotherapy is well established as the only allergen-specific and disease-modifying treatment for IgE-mediated allergies and has long-lasting effects.

In fact, more than 25% of the population suffer from IgE-mediated allergies which therefore represent a major health burden of our society, particularly because untreated allergy often progresses to severe disabling forms of disease, such as asthma and sometimes kills sensitized people through anaphylaxis.

The pathomechanisms of allergy are meanwhile quite well investigated and the disease-causing allergens are characterized in great detail down to their molecular structures. We are thus beginning to see several new strategies for allergen-specific immunotherapy on the horizon, several of which are summarized in this issue. It thus seems that hundred years after the first experimental attempts to "desensitize" hayfever patients we are now capable of developing powerful and rational forms of immunotherapy which hold promise for curing allergy sufferers and eventually may allow real prophylactic vaccination against allergy. It is thus quite possible that allergy may become eradicated similar as certain forms of infectious diseases through vaccination.

Rudolf Valenta
Robert L. Coffman

Contents

Contributors

U. Baranyi, Division of Transplantation, Department of Surgery, Vienna General Hospital, Medical University of Vienna, Vienna, Austria e-mail: Ulrike.baranyi@meduniwien.ac.at

K. Blaser, Department of Clinical Chemistry and Molecular Diagnostics, Medical Faculty, Biomedical Research Centre (BMFZ), Philipps University of Marburg, Hans-Meerwein-Str. 2, 35043, Marburg, Germany e-mail: kblaser@siaf.uzh.ch

M. L. Conrad, Department of Clinical Chemistry and Molecular Diagnostics, Medical Faculty, Biomedical Research Centre (BMFZ), Philipps University of Marburg, Hans-Meerwein-Str. 2, 35043, Marburg, Germany e-mail: Conradml@gmail.com

O. Cromwell, Allergopharma Joachim Ganzer KG, Hermann-Koerner-Strasse 52, 21465, Reinbek, Germany e-mail: oliver.cromwell@allergopharma.de

J. Edlmayr, Division of Immunopathology, Department of Pathophysiology and Allergy Research, Center for Pathophysiology, Infectiology and Immunology, Medical University of Vienna, Vienna, Austria

H. Fiebig, Allergopharma Joachim Ganzer KG, Hermann-Koerner-Strasse 52, 21465, Reinbek, Germany

S. Flicker, Division of Immunopathology, Department of Pathophysiology and Allergy Research, Center for Pathophysiology, Infectiology and Immunology, Vienna General Hospital, Medical University of Vienna, Waehringer Guertel 18-20, 1090, Vienna, Austria e-mail: sabine.flicker@meduniwien.ac.at

M. Focke-Tejkl, Christian Doppler Laboratory for Allergy Research, Medical University of Vienna, AKH Ebene 3Q, Waehringer Guertel 18–20, 1090, Vienna, Austria e-mail: margarete.focke-tejkl@meduniwien.ac.at

E. Gadermaier, Division of Immunopathology, Department of Pathophysiology and Allergy Research, Center for Pathophysiology, Infectiology and Immunology,

Vienna General Hospital, Medical University of Vienna, Waehringer Guertel 18-20, 1090, Vienna, Austria

M. Gattringer, Division of Transplantation, Department of Surgery, Vienna General Hospital, Medical University of Vienna, Vienna, Austria

A. Hofmann, Department of Pediatrics Allergy and Immunology, Duke University Medical Center, Durham, NC 27710, USA

F. Horak, ENT University Clinic, University of Vienna, Vienna, Austria

P. Johansen, Department of Dermatology, University Hospital of Zurich, 8091, Zurich, Switzerland

T. M. Kündig, Department of Dermatology, University Hospital of Zurich, 8091, Zurich, Switzerland

M. Larché, Department of Medicine, Firestone Institute for Respiratory Health, McMaster University, HSC 4H20, 1200 Main Street West, Hamilton, ON L8N 3Z5, Canada e-mail: larche@mcmaster.ca

B. Linhart, Division of Immunopathology, Department of Pathophysiology and Allergy Research, Center for Pathophysiology, Infectiology and Immunology, Medical University of Vienna, Vienna, Austria

C. Madritsch, Division of Immunopathology, Department of Pathophysiology and Allergy Research, Center for Pathophysiology, Infectiology and Immunology, Vienna General Hospital, Medical University of Vienna, Waehringer Guertel 18-20, 1090, Vienna, Austria

H. -J. Malling, Allergy Clinic 4222, National University Hospital, Blegdamsvej 9, 2100, Copenhagen, Denmark e-mail: all-unit@rh.dk

L. Mascarell, Research and Development, Stallergènes, 6 rue Alexis de Tocqueville, 92160, Antony, France

P. Moingeon, Research and Development, Stallergènes, 6 rue Alexis de Tocqueville, 92160, Antony, France

V. Niederberger, Department of Otorhinolaryngology, Medical University of Vienna, Vienna, Austria

K. Niespodziana, Division of Immunopathology, Department of Pathophysiology and Allergy Research, Center for Pathophysiology, Infectiology and Immunology, Medical University of Vienna, Vienna, Austria

G. Pauli, Faculté de médecine, Université de Strasbourg, Strasbourg, France

P. Rancitelli, Department of Pediatrics Allergy and Immunology, Ohio State University, Columbus, OH, USA

H. Renz, Department of Clinical Chemistry and Molecular Diagnostics, Medical Faculty, Biomedical Research Centre (BMFZ), Philipps University of Marburg,

Hans-Meerwein-Str. 2, 35043, Marburg, Germany e-mail: renzh@med.uni-marburg.de

G. Senti, Clinical Trials Center, Center for Clinical Research, University and University Hospital of Zurich, Rämistrasse 100, 8091, Zurich, Switzerland e-mail: gabriela.senti@usz.ch

S. Tourdot, Research and Development, Stallergènes, 6 rue Alexis de Tocqueville, 92160, Antony, France e-mail: stourdot@stallergenes.fr

R. Valenta, Christian Doppler Laboratory for Allergy Research, Medical University of Vienna, AKH Ebene 3Q, Waehringer Guertel 18–20, 1090, Vienna, Austria e-mail: rudolf.valenta@meduniwien.ac.at

L. Van Overtvelt, Research and Development, Stallergènes, 6 rue Alexis de Tocqueville, 92160, Antony, France e-mail: lvanovertvelt@stallergenes.fr

T. Wekerle, Division of Transplantation, Department of Surgery, Vienna General Hospital, Medical University of Vienna, Vienna, Austria e-mail: Thomas.Wekerle@meduniwien.ac.at

A. Wesley Burks, Department of Pediatrics Allergy and Immunology, Duke University Medical Center, Durham, NC 27710, USA e-mail: wesley.burks@duke.edu

A. Zimmer, Research and Development, Stallergènes, 6 rue Alexis de Tocqueville, 92160, Antony, France e-mail: azimmer@stallergenes.fr

Immunological Approaches for Tolerance Induction in Allergy

Melanie L. Conrad, Harald Renz and Kurt Blaser

Abstract Allergy is the consequence of an inappropriate inflammatory immune response generated against harmless environmental antigens. In allergic disorders such as asthma and rhinitis, the Th2 mediated phenotype is a result of loss of peripheral tolerance mechanisms. In cases such as these, approaches such as immunotherapy attempt to treat the underlying cause of allergic disease by restoring tolerance. Immunotherapy initiates many complex mechanisms within the immune system that result in initiation of innate immunity, activation of both cellular and humoral B cell immunity, as well as triggering T regulatory subsets which are major players in the establishment of peripheral tolerance. Though studies clearly demonstrate immunotherapy to be efficacious, research to improve this treatment is ongoing. Investigation of allergenicity versus immunogenicity, native versus modified allergens, and the use of adjuvant and modality of dosing are all current strategies for immunotherapy advancement that will be reviewed in this article.

Abbreviations

APC	Antigen presenting cell
Breg	B regulatory cell
CTLA4	Cytotoxic lymphocyte antigen 4

M. L. Conrad (✉) · H. Renz · K. Blaser
Department of Clinical Chemistry and Molecular Diagnostics, Medical Faculty,
Biomedical Research Centre (BMFZ), Philipps University of Marburg,
Hans-Meerwein-Str. 2, 35043 Marburg, Germany
e-mail: conradml@gmail.com

H. Renz
e-mail: renzh@med.uni-marburg.de

K. Blaser
e-mail: kblaser@siaf.uzh.ch

Current Topics in Microbiology and Immunology (2011) 352: 1–26
DOI: 10.1007/82_2011_128

Published Online: 20 May 2011

DC	Dendritic cell
FoxP3	Forkhead box protein 3
NLR	NOD-like receptor
PBMC	Peripheral blood mononuclear cells
PRR	Pattern recognition receptor
SCIT	Subcutaneous immotherapy
SLIT	Sublingual immunotherapy
TCR	T cell receptor
Th	T helper
iTreg	Inducible T regulatory cell
TLR	Toll-like receptor
Treg	T regulatory cell
T_R1	Type 1 T regulatory cell
tTreg	Thymus derived t regulatory cell

Contents

1 Introduction

Allergy is based on a complex dysregulation of the immune system whereby harmless environmental antigens trigger an inappropriate immune reaction. Clinically, an allergy can manifest in many different forms including local reactions such as asthma, rhinitis and skin inflammation, as well as systemic reactions to food, venom or drugs. These allergic phenotypes are complex and depend on many factors including genetic and environmental influences, the specific organs affected and the type and quantity of allergen (Larche 2006). Complicating matters further, exacerbations of current allergy are not only allergen driven but can also be brought about by infection (Tauro et al. 2008), pollutants (Riedl 2008) or non-specific stimuli (Gelardi et al. 2009).

In general, the development of an allergic response requires first that an individual be sensitized, a reaction involving the priming of specific CD4+ T-helper (Th) 2 cells, the production of the cytokine IL-4, isotype switching in B cells to produce IgE antibodies and binding of IgE antibodies to mast cells. After sensitization, secondary exposure to a specific allergen engages IgE coated mast cells which leads to mast cell degranulation and initiation of the allergic immune response. It is during secondary exposure to allergen that the complex clinical phenotype becomes apparent and it is well known that different mechanisms are responsible for the initiation of particular allergic phenotypes. For instance, patients that suffer from allergic asthma and allergic rhinitis exhibit mainly local Th2 type reactions (Pipet et al. 2009), atopic dermatitis patients exhibit an initial Th2 response that is converted to Th1 during the chronification of the disease (Leung and Bieber 2003; Novak et al. 2003; Werfel et al. 1996) and patients with food, drug and venom allergies often react by systemic anaphylaxis (Sicherer and Leung 2009). Due to the complexity of these different allergic responses, this review will concentrate specifically on two Th2 mediated allergic disorders, asthma and rhinitis (hay fever).

2 The Immune Response to Allergens is Regulated by T cells

Many immune mediators play important roles in the development of allergic disease, initiating pathways that cumulate in the differentiation of particular T cell subsets. In both healthy and diseased individuals, these subsets of effector T cells act to coordinate the entire immune system. Classically, Th cells were divided into two major subsets, Th1 and Th2, determined by cytokine profile and effector function. In the last 13 years however, T regulatory (Treg) cells have emerged as very important mediators of immune homeostasis, and are now at the forefront of research efforts. In recent years, still more T cell subtypes have been discovered such as Th17 (Burgler et al. 2009) and Th9 (Dardalhon et al. 2008a) both of which promote tissue inflammation.

The differentiation of naïve T cells to an effector subset is largely dependent on the cytokine milieu. Production of IL-12 and IFNγ by cells of the innate immune system stimulate the production of the transcription factor T-bet, Fig. 1. This results in the differentiation of Th1 cells that principally secrete IFNγ in response to intracellular pathogens. The Th2 cell lineage is generated in the presence of IL-4 due to activation of the transcription factor GATA3, Fig. 1. Th2 cells mainly utilize IL-4, IL-5 and IL-13 to regulate the clearance of extracellular

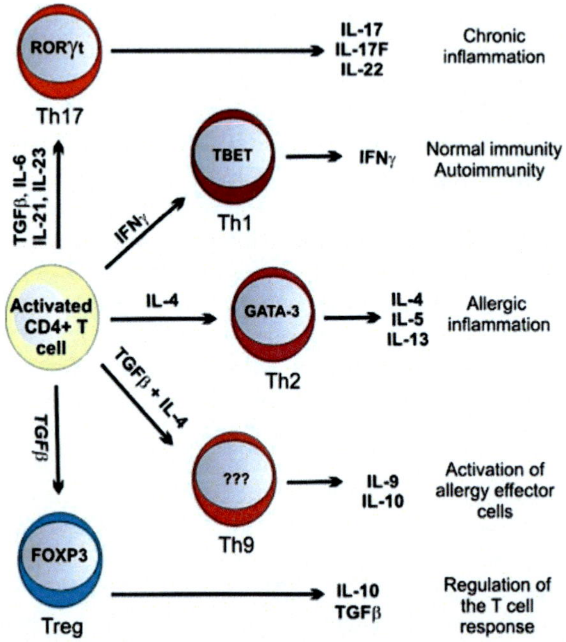

Fig. 1 Differentiation of T effector subsets from an activated CD4+ T cell

pathogens such as parasites. When a Th1 or Th2 response becomes dysregulated it leads to exaggerated inflammatory responses that are the foundation of autoimmunity and allergy, respectively (Dardalhon et al. 2008b).

Relatively new on the scene, Th17 cells are generated in the presence of both IL-6 and TGFβ; these cytokines initiate Th17 cell production by activation of the transcription factor RORγt, shown in Fig. 1. Th17 cells promote neutrophilic inflammation and appear to be responsible for eliminating both intra and extracellular pathogens through the secretion of cytokines IL-6, IL-8, IL-17A, IL-17F, IL-22, IL-26 and TNFα. Similarly to Th1 cells, an overabundance of the TH17 response leads to autoimmune disease and chronic inflammation (Schmidt-Weber et al. 2007). Finally, one of the most recent additions to the T cell subtype family is Th9. During an allergic response, the presence of IL-4 coupled with TGF-β leads to the differentiation of the Th9 cell which produces IL-9 and IL-10. Despite the abundant production of IL-10, Th9 cells do not have regulatory properties and instead act to promote tissue inflammation (Akdis and Akdis 2009; Dardalhon et al. 2008a, b; Veldhoen et al. 2008). While Th1, Th2, Th17 and Th9 subsets all generate inflammatory responses to various mediators, Treg cells act as a safeguard against unnecessary inflammation through immunosuppressive means. It is the complex interplay between these subsets that determines the health status of an individual.

Treg cells are indispensable for the maintenance of immune homeostasis and different subsets of these cells are defined by where they originate and what cytokines they secrete. Thymus derived Treg cells (tTreg, "natural" Treg), which were among the first lineage identified, are produced in the thymus, are

Table 1 Characteristics of T regulatory cell subtypes

	Thymus derived T regs	Induced T regs	
	"Natural"	TR1	Th3
Development			
Region	Thymus	Periphery	Periphery
Precursor	CD4+ precursor	CD4+CD25−	CD4+CD25−
Differentiation factors	?	IL-10, IFNα	TGFβ, IL-4
Markers			
CD4	+	+	+
CD25	+	+	+
CTLA4	+	+	+
FoxP3	+	/	+
Main mode of action	Cell contact suppression	Cytokine secretion	Cytokine secretion
Cytokines secreted			
IL-10	+	+++	+
TGF-β	+	+	+++

+ indicates expression or amount of secretion, /indicates not expressed

CD4+CD25+ and express the transcription factor forkhead box protein 3 (FoxP3), shown in Fig. 1 and Table 1 (Blaser 2008; Feuerer et al. 2009). The importance of this cell type is best exemplified by the Scurfy mouse, in which animals that fail to develop Treg cells acquire a rapidly fatal lymphoproliferative disease (Appleby and Ramsdell 2008; Brunkow et al. 2001; Khattri et al. 2001). Two additional Treg subsets, type 1 regulatory T cells (T_R1) and Th3 cells, have also been identified that can be induced in the periphery by IL-10 and TGFβ exposure, respectively, Table 1. Both tTreg cells and T_R1 cells secrete large amounts of IL-10 and TGFβ, whereas Th3 cells secrete primarily TGFβ (Workman et al. 2009).

Evidence for the regulatory capabilities of Treg cells is demonstrated by functional studies showing the suppression of both autoimmune and allergic responses by this cell type (Ozdemir et al. 2009; Walters et al. 2009). Treg cells have a major influence on both innate and adaptive immune cell types and are capable of suppressing the proliferation and differentiation of T cells as well as limiting the effector functions of B cells, NK and NK T cells, macrophages and dendritic cells (DC), shown in Fig. 2 (Ghiringhelli et al. 2005; Letourneau et al. 2009; Lim et al. 2005; Piccirillo and Shevach 2001). The role of Treg cells in the active suppression of inappropriate or excessive inflammatory responses is known as peripheral tolerance induction.

3 Tolerance

In order for the immune system to function properly there must be systems in place that allow for the discrimination of self versus non-self as well as harmless versus dangerous foreign molecules. There are several sophisticated mechanisms in the

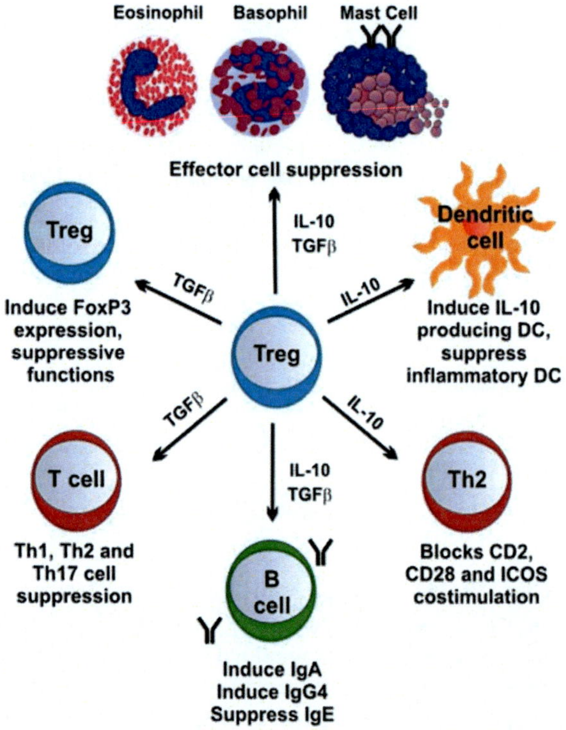

Fig. 2 The effects of Treg generated IL-10 and TGF*β* on cells of the immune system

immune system that allow this interplay to occur including clonal deletion, anergy and immunoregulation. Regarding self versus non-self determination, clonal deletion (central tolerance) acts to delete self-reactive lymphocytes during development in the bone marrow and thymus before they mature into competent immune cells (Hogquist et al. 2005; McCaughtry and Hogquist 2008). In the periphery, tolerance mechanisms such as anergy and immunoregulation allow lymphocytes to distinguish between benign and harmful antigens after T cell development (peripheral tolerance). Anergy is a state of unresponsiveness that occurs when lymphocytes recognize an antigen in the absence of a secondary, co-stimulatory signal. Continual recognition of antigen in the absence of co-stimulation eventually results in the elimination of anergic lymphocytes via activation induced cell death (Wells 2009). Immunoregulation is a second system in the maintenance of peripheral tolerance in which Treg cells play an essential role in the control of immune homeostasis. In the context of allergy, dysregulated inflammatory responses are due to a failure of the immunoregulatory mechanisms that suppress reactions to harmless substances in the periphery. Hence, inducing peripheral tolerance to the offending allergen, possibly through the alteration of the Treg response, is the ultimate goal of allergy treatment.

4 Current Treatments for Allergy

Anti-inflammatory therapy and specific immunotherapy are the two present methods used to treat allergy that work in different ways. Anti-inflammatory therapy is an allergen unspecific treatment that involves using medications such as antihistamines, anti-IgE, epinephrine or corticosteroids, alone or in combination, to block the action of allergic mediators or generally suppress the immune system (Bjermer 2008; DuBuske and Kowal 2009; Pelaia et al. 2008). Though the use of medication is presently crucial for the control of allergy, this treatment provides only temporary results. Treatments involving more permanent methods that affect the underlying cause of the allergic disorder are highly desirable.

Immunotherapy differs from anti-inflammatory therapy by attempting to affect the cause of the allergy directly by inducing peripheral immune tolerance to a particular allergen. The earliest attempts to perform immunotherapy for allergy were initiated approximately 100 years ago when, in 1911, Leonard Noon and John Freeman immunized hay fever patients with subcutaneous injections of pollen extract. Though the underlying mechanisms of allergy and immunotherapy would not begin to be discovered for many years and the strategy was erroneously based on the idea that grass pollen was toxic, successful outcomes were seen to last up to one year after cessation of treatment. (Cohen et al. 2003; Noon 1955).

In the present day, allergen specific immunotherapy is recognized as a highly specific and effective method to treat certain types of allergy. Though not generally recommended for food or drug allergies, this therapy is proving particularly effective for patients with allergic rhinitis and allergic asthma (Abramson et al. 2003; Calderon et al. 2007; Pipet et al. 2009). Immunotherapy treatments are beneficial as they target the underlying cause of the disorder with long term results; disease remission is reported to last for 3–5 years after cessation of treatment (Durham 2008). In addition to this, immunotherapy is also extremely important in preventing the progression of allergic disease, for instance from rhinitis to asthma, and stopping the further development of new sensitizations against other allergens (Des Roches et al. 1997; Jacobsen et al. 2007). Though there are many protocol variations, the general treatment method consists of multiple administrations of an allergen vaccine with concentrations that increase in a step-wise manner until the maintenance dose is reached. The maintenance dose is then continued for a minimum of three years (Didier et al. 2007; Srivastava et al. 2009). The most common type of immunotherapy in use today, subcutaneous immunotherapy (SCIT), acts by inducing peripheral tolerance to the allergen vaccine administered.

5 Tolerance Induction

In the process of becoming tolerant, the immune system is modified in many different ways. Innate immune mechanisms are activated which, in turn, trigger the generation of specific T cell subsets. The subsequent cytokine secretion from these activated T cells has wide ranging effects from reducing proinflammatory cell recruitment and activation, to modulating B cell antibody and cellular responses. Demonstrating this, many types of immune modulation have been documented after successful immunotherapy including direct suppression of antigen presenting cells (APC), induction of Treg subsets, altered IL-10 and TGFβ cytokine levels, suppression of mast cells and basophils and altered allergen specific antibody titres (Akdis et al. 1998, 2007; Francis et al. 2003).

5.1 The T Cell Response and Cytokine Secretion

Of the many T cell effector subsets, Treg cells have been acknowledged as critical players in allergy in both humans and mice. Lessons from mouse models have established the relevance of Treg cells in experimental asthma. Adoptive transfer of Treg cells into cockroach allergen sensitized and challenged mice resulted in improvement of airway reactivity and airway inflammation (McGee and Agrawal 2009). Furthermore, accumulation of Treg cells in the draining lymph nodes of mice is associated with the spontaneous resolution of chronic asthma (Carson et al. 2008). In patients with allergies such as asthma and rhinitis, accumulated evidence also suggests a strong association between allergy and a disruption of Treg cell function. Rhinitis patients have a decreased nasal FoxP3 expression compared with control subjects (Van Bruaene et al. 2008) and Treg cells from allergic subjects have a decreased ability to suppress cytokine responses in vitro (Ling et al. 2004). Dysregulated Treg cell function is associated strongly with allergy in both mouse models and human patients.

Considering immunotherapy, the induction of Treg cells is essential for the generation of immune tolerance. In adult patients who received successful immunotherapy, the frequency of FoxP3 Treg cells was increased in the nasal mucosa following SCIT with grass pollen allergen (Radulovic et al. 2008) and in PBMCs following sublingual immunotherapy (SLIT) with birch pollen allergen (Bohle et al. 2007). Upregulated Treg responses were also correlated with an increase in IL-10 expression. Interestingly, a recent pediatric study measuring the outcome of SLIT for patients treated with tree pollen allergens found correlations between FoxP3 mRNA expression and tolerance induction as well as IL-17 mRNA expression and poor therapeutic outcome (Nieminen et al. 2009). The fact that particular T cell subtypes can be associated with therapeutic outcome highlights the importance of ascertaining the mechanisms that generate T cell subtypes in successful immunotherapy.

Treg cells contribute to tolerance induction in immunotherapy both by cell–cell interactions and cytokine secretion. Concentrating for the moment on direct cellular interactions, cell contact suppression by Tregs is mediated by the constitutive expression of the cytotoxic lymphocyte antigen 4 (CTLA4). CTLA4 is a powerful suppressor of the immune response as evidenced by the lethal multi-organ inflammation observed CTLA4 knockout mice (Waterhouse et al. 1995). In the induction of peripheral tolerance, CTLA4 on allergen-activated Treg cells interacts with APCs to down modulate their expression. Illustrating this in vitro, CTLA4+FoxP3+ Treg cells out-competed DC interactions with other T cell subsets by forming aggregates around the DC. In addition to this, Treg cells were shown to downregulate APCs both in vitro and in vivo through CTLA4 dependent binding to CD80 and CD86 (Onishi et al. 2008; Wing et al. 2008).

In addition to cellular interactions, certain Treg cell subsets are known for the production of large quantities of IL-10 and TGFβ which play an important role in tolerance induction, Table 1 (Blaser and Akdis 2004). In the normal state, healthy individuals maintain subsets of allergen specific IL-10 secreting T cells at a higher frequency than both IL-4 (Th1) and IFNγ (Th2) secreting T cells (Akdis et al. 2004). In allergy, a marked reduction in IL-10 is noted in comparison with healthy subjects in both mouse models and humans. Patients with asthma have lower concentrations of IL-10 in the bronchoalveolar lavage (BAL) fluid than healthy controls (Borish et al. 1996) and a more severe asthma phenotype is associated with promoter polymorphisms in the IL-10 gene (Lim et al. 1998). Demonstrating the suppressive effects IL-10 and TGFβ, secretion of these cytokines from allergen specific T cells in non-allergic patients acted to suppress both Th1 and Th2 cytokine responses to dust mite and birch pollen allergens. In allergic patients undergoing specific immunotherapy, similar immunosuppressive effects from the CD4+CD25+ T cells were observed (Jutel et al. 2003).

IL-10 and TGFβ have established roles in the generation of peripheral tolerance, shown in Fig. 2. Originally described as a mouse Th2 factor that inhibited Th1 cytokine secretion (Fiorentino et al. 1989), IL-10 is now known to be produced by numerous cell types such as Treg cells, Th1 and Th2 lymphocytes, B lymphocytes, DCs, monocytes, macrophages, mast cells and natural killer cells (Ogawa et al. 2008). IL-10 is recognized for its powerful inhibitory effects on many cell types and the literature provides numerous examples of this in both humans and mice (Moore et al. 2001). In a mouse model of experimental asthma IL-10 administration suppressed both IL-5 production and eosinophil recruitment (Zuany-Amorim et al. 1995). In humans cells in vitro, IL-10 was shown to suppress T cell cytokine synthesis from PBMC by inhibition of CD28/B7.1 interaction (Schandene et al. 1994) and modulate antibody production by inhibiting IgE and enhancing IgG4 (Punnonen et al. 1993; Satoguina et al. 2005). These inhibitory effects coupled with the strong association of IL-10 secretion with allergen tolerance induced by immunotherapy illustrates the importance of this cytokine. TGFβ is an essential cytokine in the maintenance of the Treg population. In mice it is required for the proliferation and suppressive actions of Treg cells (Huber et al. 2004), as well as for the peripheral induction of CD4+CD25− cells to a FoxP3+CD4+CD25+ subtype, shown in Table 1 (Chen et al. 2003). As a suppressive cytokine in human immunotherapy, TGFβ affects T cell proliferation, differentiation and apoptosis. Additionally, both IL-10 and TGFβ have the ability to down regulate MHC II expression and suppress costimulatory molecules on APCs (Jutel et al. 2003). Secretion of IL-10 and TGFβ from Treg cells as well as direct cell–cell interactions are essential for peripheral tolerance and are heavily involved in successful immunotherapy treatment (Workman et al. 2009).

5.2 Histamine and Histamine Receptors in Tolerance Induction

Histamine is a pharmacologically active mediator secreted from effector cells during allergic inflammation. Of the four different histamine receptors (HR1, HR2, HR3 and HR4), HR1 and HR2 are expressed on activated effector T cells (Jutel et al. 2001, 2002). Human CD4+Th1 cells predominantly express the HR1 whereas Th2 cells predominantly display the HR2. This differential expression of HR1 and HR2 results in a differential regulation of the allergic response by histamine. (Jutel et al. 2001, 2002). In this regulatory process, histamine induces the production of IL-10 by DCs (Mazzoni et al. 2001) and Th2 cells (Osna et al. 2001) as well as enhancing the suppressive activity of TGFβ secreted by T cells (Kunzmann et al. 2003). These regulatory effects which suppress IL-4 and IL-13 production as well as T cell proliferation, are mediated via the HR2 mostly expressed on Th2 cells. (Jutel et al. 2001). Thus, HR2 up-regulation on allergen specific Th2 cells increases IL-10 and TGFβ production and regulatory activity and suppresses the allergen-stimulated Th2 response. Accordingly, histamine and its HR2, participates in feedback- and fine-regulation of the allergic immune response and of peripheral tolerance induction.

5.3 B Cells in Tolerance Induction

Though normally thought of as pathogenic when referring to allergy, B cells also play a positive role in immunotherapy. Accordingly, the production of allergen specific IgG4 during successful immunotherapy is proposed to play a major role in tolerance induction. In certain patients, levels of IgG4 in patients reflect allergen exposure, increase in a dose dependent manner, are highly stable during the long immunotherapy time period and appear to protect against allergy (Peng et al. 1992; Rossi et al. 2007). The protective phenotype associated with the emergence of allergen specific IgG4 antibodies includes a reduction in mast cells, basophils and inflammatory mediators, as well as prevention of IgE mediated allergen presentation to T cells (Mobs et al. 2008; Strait et al. 2006). It has been proposed that IgG4 acts as either a blocking antibody that competes for IgE binding sites (Flicker et al. 2002; Jackola et al. 2002; van Neerven et al. 1999) or acts via the binding of IgG4-allergen complexes to the FcγRIIB receptors on mast cells to induce a deactivation signal (Daeron et al. 1995; Pipet et al. 2009).

In some patients treated successfully with immunotherapy, marked changes are observed in the allergen specific antibody composition. After an initial, transient increase in serum specific IgE, levels of this antibody decrease over months and years of treatment (Fennerty et al. 1988; Van Ree et al. 1997). Together with decreases in IgE levels, allergen specific IgG4 antibodies are observed to increase throughout the treatment period (Mobs et al. 2008; Wachholz et al. 2003). Demonstrating the clinical importance of allergen specific antibody isotypes, IgG4 concentrations or ratios of IgG4:IgG_{total} and IgE:IgG4 may be used as an indicator of treatment efficacy and tolerance induction (Aalberse et al. 2009; Nouri-Aria et al. 2004). However, due to large variances in antibody production in individual patients, IgG4 antibody levels cannot be used as a predictable marker for successful immunotherapy in the individual patient (Jeannin et al. 1994). Future research into individual IgG4 antibody production may shed light into how this isotype plays a role in tolerance induction and help to identify traits in individuals that are likely to activate IgG4 production.

In addition to antibody production, B cells may also play an antibody-independent role in the induction of peripheral tolerance. Evidence for this is seen in a mouse model of tolerance to aeroallergens in which the presence of allergen specific B cells in BCR transgenic mice resulted in enhancement of CD4+ T cell tolerance to intranasally applied allergen. This regulation by B cells occurred in an antibody-independent manner. In contrast, tolerance was not achievable in B cell deficient mice (Tsitoura et al. 2002). Due to the antibody-independent nature of this response, it is hypothesized that different B cell subsets may play an immunoregulatory role through either cytokine secretion or cell contact mechanisms. B cells with suppressive capabilities, dubbed B regulatory cells (Breg), are specifically induced under inflammatory conditions and are capable of contributing to tolerance mechanisms (Mizoguchi and Bhan 2006).

B cells with regulatory capabilities were first recognized in 1974 with the demonstration of B cell mediated suppression of delayed type sensitivity reactions in guinea pigs (Katz et al. 1974; Neta and Salvin 1974). Though the majority of Breg cell studies are currently investigating autoimmunity (Manjarrez-Orduno et al. 2009) recent studies in allergy associate B cell secretion of IL-10 and TGFβ with suppressive capabilities (Mizoguchi and Bhan 2006). When stimulated in vitro by immunotherapy extracts, human B cells secrete high amounts of IL-10, which act to suppress IL-4 mediated IgE expression (Milovanovic et al. 2009). In a mouse model of ovalbumin induced experimental asthma, adoptive transfer of B cells into sensitized mice attenuated the resulting allergic airway disease through migration to local inflammatory sites and TGFβ mediated conversion of CD4+CD45− effector T cells to CD4+CD25+FoxP3+ Treg cells (Singh et al. 2008). The involvement of Breg cells in immunotherapy provides an interesting new avenue for exploration in allergy and immunotherapy as an additional system that contributes to tolerance induction.

5.4 Innate Immunity and Tolerance Induction

As natural allergen extracts applied in immunotherapy may also contain components such as lipopolysaccharide, saccharides and nucleic acids, immunotherapy treatments can also have a non-allergen specific effect. These non-allergenic molecules contain pathogen associated molecular patterns (PAMPs) that activate innate immune cells through pattern recognition receptors (PRR) in the Toll-like receptor (TLR) or NOD-like receptor (NLR) families. Initiation of the immune system by PAMPS generates particular antigen presenting cell subtypes which subsequently results in co-stimulation and production of beneficial T cell subsets such as Treg cells. The generation of Treg cells thus contributes to the suppression of the allergic phenotype (Pipet et al. 2009). Examples of innate immune stimulation in patients undergoing SCIT include IL-10 production by monocytes and macrophages (Nouri-Aria et al. 2004), and a mouse model of oral tolerance has identified TGFβ expressing DC subsets that induce functional FoxP3+ Treg cells from FoxP3− cells in the periphery (Yamazaki and Steinman 2009).

6 Improving Current Immunotherapy Strategies

The goal of immunotherapy is to induce peripheral immune tolerance to specific allergens while maintaining safety and tolerability for the patient (Schmidt-Weber and Blaser 2005). While clinical studies indicate that with strict adherence to guidelines, SCIT is relatively well tolerated, alternative methods to induce tolerance while reducing the risk of adverse events and simplifying the protocol for patient compliance, continue to be investigated (Pipet et al. 2009). A number of considerations such as the type of allergen, the modality and the use of adjuvant all represent potential targets for the advancement of immunotherapy.

6.1 Allergen: Immunogenicity and Allergenicity

Focusing on allergens, tolerance induction may be dependent on both the immunogenicity and allergenicity of the vaccine used for immunotherapy. Immunogenicity is defined as the capacity of a vaccine to induce a beneficial immune response, whereas allergenicity is the potential to cause an allergic reaction. The immunogenicity and allergenicity of a molecule are defined by specific epitopes present on the macromolecule. B cell epitopes, which are specifically recognized by antibodies, are located on the three dimensional structure of the antigen molecule whereas T cell epitopes must be first phagocytosed by an APC and presented in the context of an MHC class II molecule on the cell surface. T cell epitopes usually consist of 8–11 linearly arranged amino acids and are specifically recognized by the T cell receptor. During an immune response, activation through a B cell epitope results in antibody class switching, whereas activation of a T cell epitope stimulates the production of T cell subsets that act to regulate the immune response. While it is not known exactly how the expression of particular epitopes shapes the immune response, it is hypothesized that the epitope profile, and thus the particular type of allergen used in vaccination, is of great importance in the induction of peripheral tolerance (Pomes 2008; Szalai et al. 2008).

Table 2 Summary of the different types of allergen used for specific immunotherapy

Allergen class	Treatment	Result
Natural	Extract from natural sources	Multiple allergens and naturally occurring substances
Chemical	Chemical—formaldehyde/ gluteraldehyde	High molecular weight allergen polymer—linked through lysine residues
	Chemical—carbamylation	Low molecular weight allergen—lysines modified to ureido groups
Recombinant	Peptide production	Generation of specific T cell epitopes only
	Intact major allergen	Recombinant whole protein allergen
	Intact hypoallergenic allergen	Recombinant whole protein allergen that mimics naturally occurring allergen isoforms with low IgE binding capacity
	Fragmentation	Fragmentation of allergen tertiary structure results in loss of B cell epitopes
	Amalgamation	Creation of allergen dimers and trimers using cDNA and expression plasmids

6.2 Type of Allergen

In an attempt to improve immunotherapy, many investigations have been aimed at modifying the allergen vaccine to reduce allergenicity while maintaining the immunogenicity and, thus, allow for successful treatment. Of the major classifications of allergens for use in immunotherapy, native, chemically modified and recombinant allergens, summarized in Table 2, will be discussed further in this section.

6.2.1 Native Allergens

Traditionally in immunotherapy, the allergen used for treatment is obtained from 'native' extracts purified from natural sources. One drawback of native allergen use is the difficulty of standardizing production. Indeed, recent studies have found significant concentration variances in birch pollen allergen preparations (Focke et al. 2009) as well as the presence of unrelated allergens (van der Veen et al. 1996) which can be problematic due to the possibility of patients developing new IgE reactivities (Moverare et al. 2002; Pauli et al. 2008). Other studies investigating native allergen extracts have found contamination in the form of endotoxin (Trivedi et al. 2003) and beta glucans (Finkelman et al. 2006), though the possible adjuvant effects of these 'contaminating' molecules are not fully understood and must be researched further. Though addressing the aforementioned concerns and developing a global standard for native allergen extract preparation are essential, further research into modified and/or recombinant allergens will provide alternative concepts to improve the allergen vaccines used in immunotherapy.

6.2.2 'Allergoid': Chemically Modified Allergens

One of the first attempts to modify allergen for use in immunotherapy was to chemically modify naturally extracted allergens by treatment with dilute formaldehyde. Today it is known that chemical modification of an allergen with formaldehyde or glutaraldehyde acts to create a high molecular weight allergen polymer by linking the amine groups from exposed lysines. Creation of allergen polymers by this method maintains immunogenicity while strongly reducing the IgE binding capability (Kahlert et al. 2000). In addition to high molecular weight allergen polymers produced by formaldehyde/glutaraldehyde treatment, treatment of allergens by carbamylation produces low molecular weight allergens that can, for example, be easily absorbed through mucosal surfaces. Carbamylation acts by transforming the N-terminus of lysine residues to a ureido group which functionally reduces allergenicity of the protein molecule (Mistrello et al. 1996; Velickovic and Jankov 2008). Successful use of chemical modification of an allergen vaccine was first performed by Marsh et al. in 1970 and allergoid vaccines have since been successfully tested in immunotherapy in both adults and children (Keskin et al. 2006; La Grutta et al. 2007; Palma-Carlos et al. 2006; Williams et al. 2007).

6.2.3 Recombinant Allergens

Yet another approach for the creation of safer immunotherapy vaccines is the production of recombinant allergens such as peptides, recombinant protein, recombinant hypoallergenic protein, allergen fragments and oligomers. Before discussing these alternatives, however, it must be considered whether single recombinant allergens can indeed mimic native allergen extracts. The fact that native allergen extracts contain a large compliment of different molecules and that there exists a virtually limitless range of potential allergens in the environment, engenders the question of whether a limited number of representative recombinant allergens can induce tolerance across a spectrum (Vrtala 2008). Studies investigating the diagnostic capabilities of recombinant allergens have found, for example, that of the six main grass pollen allergens, a panel of four was able to diagnose grass pollen allergy in all patients tested (Laffer et al. 1996; Valenta et al. 1998; Vrtala et al. 1993). Consequently, it appears that of all allergenic possibilities, a few major allergens can determine the susceptibility of many.

Using recombinant technology it is possible to generate peptides containing short, linear, allergen-derived T cell epitopes for use in immunotherapy to specifically target CD4+ T cells. The process involves screening for T cell activity after stimulation with overlapping synthetic peptides that span the known allergen molecule sequence (Akdis and Blaser 2000). Due to their small size and lack of secondary and tertiary structures, peptide sequences have a reduced ability to bind IgE and thus have greatly reduced allergenicity. Murine studies have demonstrated the effectiveness of peptide immunotherapy in inducing tolerance to a mite allergen *Der p 1* (Hoyne et al. 1993) and a cat allergen *Fel d 1* (Briner et al. 1993). Clinically, the allergens *Fel d 1*, bee venom *Api m 1* and ragweed *Amb a 1* have been heavily researched in humans. Although initial clinical trials using *Fel d 1* peptide immunotherapy demonstrated positive effects in patients with asthma, treatment also induced numerous adverse effects that were later attributed to the peptide length and high dosage (Larche 2007). More recent trials with *Fel d 1* have managed to achieve tolerance induction with greatly reduced adverse events through the use of shorter peptides and reduced doses (Alexander et al. 2005; Verhoef et al. 2005), however much research is still required to determine the optimal dosing, timing and route for peptide immunotherapy.

The use of recombinant whole protein and fragmented allergens are also being investigated for immunotherapy improvement. Considering for the moment whole protein, initial clinical trials have found recombinant major grass pollen (Jutel et al. 2005) and birch pollen allergens (Pauli et al. 2008) to be effective for immunotherapy treatment. Moreover, comparison of clinical studies using either recombinant allergen or native allergen extract revealed similar efficacy in both of these treatments (Kahler et al. 1999; Pauli et al. 2008). In addition to recombinant major allergens, there has also been recent interest in the generation of hypoallergenic allergens. Hypoallergenic allergens are naturally occurring isoforms of a particular allergen that have reduced IgE reactivity while maintaining T cell epitope recognition. It is hypothesized that the use of recombinant hypoallergenic isoforms can further reduce adverse events generated by immunotherapy due to the greatly reduced allergenicity of the protein. Current research has revealed hypoallergenic isoforms of birch pollen *Bet v 1* (Wagner et al. 2008) mite *Blo t 12* (Zakzuk et al. 2009) and *Der p 1* (Walgraffe et al. 2009) that may be beneficial for use in future allergen vaccines.

Recombinant technology offers many techniques for the generation of new allergen vaccines. While peptides and whole protein allergens continue to be investigated, engineered fragments of allergen also provide a promising avenue for exploration. Fragmentation reduces the allergenicity of a protein molecule since during the process one or more major B cell epitopes are removed from the tertiary structure. Illustrating this concept, *Bet v 1* birch pollen allergen fragments have been engineered that promote tolerogenic responses in both mice and rabbits (Vrtala et al. 2000). Finally, just as fragments of allergen have reduced allergenicity, allergen multimers also contain fewer B cell epitopes. Allergen dimers and trimers that are genetically engineered using cDNA subunits and expression plasmids are also being studied for use in immunotherapy. Demonstrating the functionality of multimeric allergen molecules, *Bet v 1* dimers and trimers stimulate T cell activity in PBMCs from allergic individuals, and have strongly reduced anaphylactic activity as observed by basophil histamine release and skin prick testing (van Hage-Hamsten et al. 1999; Vrtala et al. 1999).

The use of recombinant allergens has a great deal of potential for the improvement of allergen vaccines. Due to the many types of recombinant technologies available, allergens can be modified in numerous ways to potentially reduce allergenicity while inducing tolerance. Though many advancements have been made in the creation of novel allergen vaccines, much research is still required to reach the full potential of recombinant allergens in the clinical setting. Through rigorous testing and understanding of the mechanisms of tolerance induction it is possible to improve immunotherapy by the use of recombinant allergens.

6.3 Modality: Route of Dosing

Since the discovery of immunotherapy, the subcutaneous route of application has been the gold standard. In an attempt to counter some of the adverse reactions that accompany SCIT, SLIT (consisting of absorption of an allergen solution or tablet through the mucosal layers under the tongue) was developed as an alternative. Considering that pediatric patients are a major group of candidates for allergy therapy, SLIT is an appealing alternative due to the simpler dosing route and the possibility of fewer clinic visits for treatment (Halken et al. 2008). Meta-analysis of SLIT in adults revealed safety and efficacy mainly for allergic rhinitis (Compalati et al. 2009; Wilson et al. 2005), however, due to current controversy in the literature over the efficacy of SLIT for children, the results of more studies must be published before conclusive decisions can be made (Campbell 2009; Halken et al. 2008; Larenas-Linnemann 2009; van Wijk 2008). SLIT is now accepted to be significantly safer than SCIT as there have been only few case reports of anaphylactic reactions (Moingeon et al. 2006) however, there is cause for caution when treating patients with SLIT that have previously discontinued SCIT due to adverse reactions (Cochard and Eigenmann 2009).

Though SLIT is an effective alternative to SCIT under these considerations, generating further knowledge regarding its mechanism of action will provide opportunities for improved second generation vaccines. Comparison of successful SLIT and SCIT treatments reveals that though both treatments generate peripheral tolerance via the induction of regulatory T cells, the manner of tolerance induction is highly dependent on the draining lymph nodes at the site of antigen application. At sites of oral immunization for SLIT, allergen is captured by Langerhans-like DCs which subsequently upregulate the expression of adhesion and trafficking receptors such as CCR7 and migrate to the mucosal draining lymph nodes (internal jugular, superficial cervical and submaxillary) in the mucosa-associated axis (Kraal et al. 2006; Moingeon et al. 2006).

While SCIT relies on introduction of allergen to sites under the skin, SLIT takes advantage of already existing oral tolerance mechanisms that are present to ensure immune tolerance to food and commensal bacteria. Lymph nodes near mucosal sites maintain a particular microenvironment that is favorable for tolerance induction. Illustrating this, murine studies show a preferential generation of "blocking" IgG2b antibodies and higher antibody responses in mucosal lymph nodes than lymph nodes near subcutaneous sites of injection (Aoyama-Kondo et al. 1992; van Helvoort et al. 2004). Though there is still much work to be done to elucidate the mechanism of SLIT, it is hypothesized to involve B cell dependent generation of Treg cells and subsequent T effector cell suppression, as well as a B cell independent development of Foxp3-LAP+TGFβ+Tregs (Sun et al. 2008).

In comparison with SCIT, one immediate drawback of SLIT is the need for 50–100 times higher allergen concentration which over time can greatly add to the cost of treatment. One of the possible explanations for this is that SCIT protocols routinely use an adjuvant as part of the vaccination regimen whereas SLIT treatment protocols do not. The use of adjuvants for immunotherapy is important for protocol improvement and many studies are testing adjuvants currently in use as well as new candidate mucosal adjuvants for future immunotherapy trials (Moingeon et al. 2006).

6.4 Adjuvant

As mentioned previously, SCIT treatment often utilizes the adjuvant aluminum hydroxide (alum) as an adsorbant and immunostimulant. Consequently, the emergence of novel immunotherapy techniques such as use of recombinant allergens (which are less potent immune stimulators than allergen extracts) and sublingual allergen application has generated a parallel search for mucosal adjuvants that can enhance the peripheral tolerance mechanisms induced during SLIT (Goldman 2008). In a murine model of SLIT using the allergen ovalbumin in conjunction with the adjuvant cholera toxin B (CTB), Sun et al. found an increased expression of FoxP3+CD25+CD4+ Treg cells in the draining lymph nodes; CTB application also greatly reduced the amount of allergen needed to elicit this effect (Sun et al. 2006). TLR ligands are also being studied as potential adjuvants due to their ability to activiate IL-10 secreting DCs that are likely to promote the emergence of Tregs. Studies by Lombardi et al. demonstrate that the application of the TLR2 ligand, Pam3CSK4 promotes the differentiation of IFNγ and IL-10 secreting CD4+ T cells both in vitro in cell culture and in vivo in a murine experimental asthma model in which mice were treated sublingually with both allergen and Pam3CSK4 (Lombardi et al. 2008). Due to the specialized micro-environments of the mucosal lymph nodes and the efficacy of SLIT, the generation of mucosal adjuvants provides a promising area for the creation of second generation SLIT vaccines.

7 Future Perspectives

Immunotherapy is a highly effective method of treating allergies such as asthma and rhinitis by inducing allergen specific tolerance in the periphery. Notwithstanding, the subject of allergy prevention by non-specific tolerance induction is also a topic of intense interest. Epidemiological findings demonstrate that certain environmental exposures such as unhygienic contact with older siblings and growing up in a farming environment may confer protection against certain allergies (Strachan 1989, 2000; von Mutius and Radon 2008). Observations from epidemiological studies lead to the formation of the hygiene hypothesis by Strachan in 1989 which basically states that exposure to microbes either prenatally or early in life may reduce the risk of developing allergies.

In addition to the great deal of epidemiological evidence supporting the hygiene hypothesis (Douwes et al. 2007; Kiechl-Kohlendorfer et al. 2007; Matheson et al. 2009; Seiskari et al. 2007), proof of concept has also been shown in animal models. In a prevention model, protective effects against murine experimental asthma were seen with both *Lactococcus* and *Acinetobacter* bacterial strains isolated from farm sites (Debarry et al. 2007), lipopolysaccharide (Lundy et al. 2003) and *Mycobacterium vaccae* (Yazi et al. 2007). Furthermore, microbes applied prenatally were also shown to have asthma preventative effects in offspring; the mechanism of which was demonstrated to be fully dependent on functional maternal TLRs (Blümer et al. 2007; Conrad et al. 2009). Though research into the mechanisms of non-specific tolerance induction and the hygiene hypothesis is still in its infancy, this subject will surely garner much interest in the years to come.

8 Conclusion

Allergy is the consequence of an inappropriate inflammatory immune response generated against harmless environmental antigens. Characterized by Th2 cytokine secretion and the production of allergen specific IgE antibodies, this type of immune reaction is the result of an imbalance between different T cell subsets, namely a reduced presence of Treg cells. Of the different methods to treat allergy, immunotherapy is a specific, highly effective means of treating allergic asthma and rhinitis that is shown to have long lasting effects after cessation of the therapy. Immunotherapy acts by initiating peripheral tolerance mechanisms and thus functions to correct the underlying pathomechanisms of allergic disease.

Though allergen immunotherapy is an effective method to treat certain allergies, there is currently much interest in improving the allergen vaccines used for treatment. Experimentation with chemical allergen modification as well as the generation of recombinant allergen proteins and peptides represent exciting new methods to improve treatment. Furthermore, testing of the route of allergen vaccine application and stimulation of the immune system by specific adjuvants may also reveal novel methods for allergen application. As more is learned about the mechanisms of tolerance induction and the improvement of allergen vaccines, we approach a better understanding of treating the underlying causes of allergy.

References

Aalberse RC, Stapel SO, Schuurman J, Rispens T (2009) Immunoglobulin G4: an odd antibody. Clin Exp Allergy 39:469–477

Abramson MJ, Puy RM, Weiner JM (2003) Allergen immunotherapy for asthma. Cochrane Database Syst Rev 4:CD001186

Akdis M, Akdis CA (2007) Mechanisms of allergen-specific immunotherapy. J Allergy Clin Immunol 119:780–791

Akdis CA, Akdis M (2009) Mechanisms and treatment of allergic disease in the big picture of regulatory T cells. J Allergy Clin Immunol 123:735–748

Akdis CA, Blaser K (2000) Regulation of specific immune responses by chemical and structural modifications of allergens. Int Arch Allergy Immunol 121:261–269

Akdis CA, Blesken T, Akdis M, Wuthrich B, Blaser K (1998) Role of interleukin 10 in specific immunotherapy. J Clin Invest 102:98–106

Akdis M, Verhagen J, Taylor A, Karamloo F, Karagiannidis C, Crameri R, Thunberg S, Deniz G, Valenta R, Fiebig H, Kegel C, Disch R, Schmidt-Weber CB, Blaser K, Akdis CA (2004) Immune responses in healthy and allergic individuals are characterized by a fine balance between allergen-specific T regulatory 1 and T helper 2 cells. J Exp Med 199:1567–1575

Alexander C, Tarzi M, Larche M, Kay AB (2005) The effect of Fel d 1-derived T-cell peptides on upper and lower airway outcome measurements in cat-allergic subjects. Allergy 60: 1269–1274

Aoyama-Kondo T, Yoshida T, Tsobe K, Nakayama A, Asai J, Oka T, Nakashima I (1992) Characterization of antibody responses of local lymph nodes to antigen given under the oral submucosa. Immunobiology 184:372–383

Appleby MW, Ramsdell F (2008) Scurfy, the Foxp3 locus, and the molecular basis of peripheral tolerance. Curr Top Microbiol Immunol 321:151–168

Bjermer L (2008) Evaluating combination therapies for asthma: pros, cons, and comparative benefits. Ther Adv Respir Dis 2:149–161

Blaser K (2008) Role of T-cell subtypes in allergic inflammations. Chem Immunol Allergy 94: xi–xv

Blaser K, Akdis CA (2004) Interleukin-10, T regulatory cells and specific allergy treatment. Clin Exp Allergy 34:328–331

Blümer N, Sel S, Virna S, Patrascan CC, Zimmermann S, Herz U, Renz H, Garn H (2007) Perinatal maternal application of *Lactobacillus rhamnosus* GG suppresses allergic airway inflammation in mouse offspring. Clin Exp Allergy 37:348–357

Bohle B, Kinaciyan T, Gerstmayr M, Radakovics A, Jahn-Schmid B, Ebner C (2007) Sublingual immunotherapy induces IL-10-producing T regulatory cells, allergen-specific T-cell tolerance, and immune deviation. J Allergy Clin Immunol 120:707–713

Borish L, Aarons A, Rumbyrt J, Cvietusa P, Negri J, Wenzel S (1996) Interleukin-10 regulation in normal subjects and patients with asthma. J Allergy Clin Immunol 97:1288–1296

Briner TJ, Kuo MC, Keating KM, Rogers BL, Greenstein JL (1993) Peripheral T-cell tolerance induced in naive and primed mice by subcutaneous injection of peptides from the major cat allergen Fel d I. Proc Natl Acad Sci USA 90:7608–7612

Brunkow ME, Jeffery EW, Hjerrild KA, Paeper B, Clark LB, Yasayko SA, Wilkinson JE, Galas D, Ziegler SF, Ramsdell F (2001) Disruption of a new forkhead/winged-helix protein, scurfin, results in the fatal lymphoproliferative disorder of the scurfy mouse. Nat Genet 27:68–73

Burgler S, Ouaked N, Bassin C, Basinski TM, Mantel PY, Siegmund K, Meyer N, Akdis CA, Schmidt-Weber CB (2009) Differentiation and functional analysis of human T(H)17 cells. J Allergy Clin Immunol 123:588–595, 595 e581–587

Calderon MA, Alves B, Jacobson M, Hurwitz B, Sheikh A, Durham S (2007) Allergen injection immunotherapy for seasonal allergic rhinitis. Cochrane Database Syst Rev 1:CD001936

Campbell DE (2009) Sublingual immunotherapy for children: are we there yet? Defining its role in clinical practice. Paediatr Respir Rev 10:69–74 quiz 74

Carson WF IV, Guernsey LA, Singh A, Vella AT, Schramm CM, Thrall RS (2008) Accumulation of regulatory T cells in local draining lymph nodes of the lung correlates with spontaneous resolution of chronic asthma in a murine model. Int Arch Allergy Immunol 145:231–243

Chen W, Jin W, Hardegen N, Lei KJ, Li L, Marinos N, McGrady G, Wahl SM (2003) Conversion of peripheral CD4+CD25− naive T cells to CD4+CD25+ regulatory T cells by TGF-beta induction of transcription factor Foxp3. J Exp Med 198:1875–1886

Cochard MM, Eigenmann PA (2009) Sublingual immunotherapy is not always a safe alternative to subcutaneous immunotherapy. J Allergy Clin Immunol 124:378–379

Cohen SG, Frankland AW, Dworetzky M (2003) Noon and Freeman on prophylactic inoculation against hay fever. J Allergy Clin Immunol 111:1142–1150

Compalati E, Penagos M, Tarantini F, Passalacqua G, Canonica GW (2009) Specific immunotherapy for respiratory allergy: state of the art according to current meta-analyses. Ann Allergy Asthma Immunol 102:22–28

Conrad ML, Ferstl R, Teich R, Brand S, Blümer N, Yildirim AO, Patrascan CC, Hanuszkiewicz A, Akira S, Wagner H, Holst O, von Mutius E, Pfefferle PI, Kirschning CJ, Garn H, Renz H (2009) Maternal TLR signaling is required for prenatal asthma protection by the nonpathogenic microbe Acinetobacter lwoffii F78. J Exp Med 206:2869–2877

Daeron M, Malbec O, Latour S, Arock M, Fridman WH (1995) Regulation of high-affinity IgE receptor-mediated mast cell activation by murine low-affinity IgG receptors. J Clin Invest 95:577–585

Dardalhon V, Awasthi A, Kwon H, Galileos G, Gao W, Sobel RA, Mitsdoerffer M, Strom TB, Elyaman W, Ho IC, Khoury S, Oukka M, Kuchroo VK (2008a) IL-4 inhibits TGF-beta-induced Foxp3+T cells and, together with TGF-beta, generates IL-9+IL-10+Foxp3(-) effector T cells. Nat Immunol 9:1347–1355

Dardalhon V, Korn T, Kuchroo VK, Anderson AC (2008b) Role of Th1 and Th17 cells in organ-specific autoimmunity. J Autoimmun 31:252–256

Debarry J, Garn H, Hanuszkiewicz A, Dickgreber N, Blümer N, von Mutius E, Bufe A, Gatermann S, Renz H, Holst O, Heine H (2007) *Acinetobacter lwoffii* and *Lactococcus lactis* strains isolated from farm cowsheds possess strong allergy-protective properties. J Allergy Clin Immunol 119:1514–1521

Des Roches A, Paradis L, Menardo JL, Bouges S, Daures JP, Bousquet J (1997) Immunotherapy with a standardized Dermatophagoides pteronyssinus extract. VI. Specific immunotherapy prevents the onset of new sensitizations in children. J Allergy Clin Immunol 99:450–453

Didier A, Malling HJ, Worm M, Horak F, Jager S, Montagut A, Andre C, de Beaumont O, Melac M (2007) Optimal dose, efficacy, and safety of once-daily sublingual immunotherapy with a 5-grass pollen tablet for seasonal allergic rhinitis. J Allergy Clin Immunol 120:1338–1345

Douwes J, Travier N, Huang K, Cheng S, McKenzie J, Le Gros G, von Mutius E, Pearce N (2007) Lifelong farm exposure may strongly reduce the risk of asthma in adults. Allergy 62: 1158–1165

DuBuske L, Kowal K (2009) Update on prescription and over-the-counter histamine inverse agonists in rhinitis therapy. Curr Allergy Asthma Rep 9:140–148

Durham SR (2008) Sublingual immunotherapy: what have we learnt from the 'big trials'? Curr Opin Allergy Clin Immunol 8:577–584

Fennerty AG, Jones KP, Davies BH, Fifield R, Edwards J (1988) Immunological changes associated with a successful outcome of pollen immunotherapy. Allergy 43:415–419

Feuerer M, Hill JA, Mathis D, Benoist C (2009) Foxp3+ regulatory T cells: differentiation, specification, subphenotypes. Nat Immunol 10:689–695

Finkelman MA, Lempitski SJ, Slater JE (2006) beta-Glucans in standardized allergen extracts. J Endotoxin Res 12:241–245

Fiorentino DF, Bond MW, Mosmann TR (1989) Two types of mouse T helper cell. IV. Th2 clones secrete a factor that inhibits cytokine production by Th1 clones. J Exp Med 170: 2081–2095

Flicker S, Steinberger P, Norderhaug L, Sperr WR, Majlesi Y, Valent P, Kraft D, Valenta R (2002) Conversion of grass pollen allergen-specific human IgE into a protective IgG(1) antibody. Eur J Immunol 32:2156–2162

Focke M, Marth K, Valenta R (2009) Molecular composition and biological activity of commercial birch pollen allergen extracts. Eur J Clin Invest 39:429–436

Francis JN, Till SJ, Durham SR (2003) Induction of IL-10+CD4+CD25+ T cells by grass pollen immunotherapy. J Allergy Clin Immunol 111:1255–1261

Gelardi M, Russo C, Fiorella ML, Fiorella R, Canonica GW, Passalacqua G (2009) When allergic rhinitis is not only allergic. Am J Rhinol Allergy 23:312–315

Ghiringhelli F, Menard C, Terme M, Flament C, Taieb J, Chaput N, Puig PE, Novault S, Escudier B, Vivier E, Lecesne A, Robert C, Blay JY, Bernard J, Caillat-Zucman S, Freitas A, Tursz T, Wagner-Ballon O, Capron C, Vainchencker W, Martin F, Zitvogel L (2005) CD4+CD25+ regulatory T cells inhibit natural killer cell functions in a transforming growth factor-beta-dependent manner. J Exp Med 202:1075–1085

Goldman M (2008) Sublingual immunotherapy: the quest for innovative adjuvants. Clin Exp Allergy 38:1705–1706

Halken S, Lau S, Valovirta E (2008) New visions in specific immunotherapy in children: an iPAC summary and future trends. Pediatr Allergy Immunol 19(Suppl 19):60–70

Hogquist KA, Baldwin TA, Jameson SC (2005) Central tolerance: learning self-control in the thymus. Nat Rev Immunol 5:772–782

Hoyne GF, O'Hehir RE, Wraith DC, Thomas WR, Lamb JR (1993) Inhibition of T cell and antibody responses to house dust mite allergen by inhalation of the dominant T cell epitope in naive and sensitized mice. J Exp Med 178:1783–1788

Huber S, Schramm C, Lehr HA, Mann A, Schmitt S, Becker C, Protschka M, Galle PR, Neurath MF, Blessing M (2004) Cutting edge: TGF-beta signaling is required for the in vivo expansion and immunosuppressive capacity of regulatory CD4+CD25+ T cells. J Immunol 173: 6526–6531

Jackola DR, Pierson-Mullany LK, Liebeler CL, Blumenthal MN, Rosenberg A (2002) Variable binding affinities for allergen suggest a 'selective competition' among immunoglobulins in atopic and non-atopic humans. Mol Immunol 39:367–377

Jacobsen L, Niggemann B, Dreborg S, Ferdousi HA, Halken S, Host A, Koivikko A, Norberg LA, Valovirta E, Wahn U, Moller C (2007) Specific immunotherapy has long-term preventive effect of seasonal and perennial asthma: 10-year follow-up on the PAT study. Allergy 62: 943–948

Jeannin P, Delneste Y, Tillie-Leblond I, Wallaert B, carlier A, Pestel J, Tonnel AB (1994) Abnormal IgG4 antibody response to aeroallergens in allergic patients. Int Arch Allergy Immunol 104:191–198

Jutel M, Watanabe T, Klunker S, Akdis M, Thomet OA, Malolepszy J, Zak-Nejmark T, Koga R, Kobayashi T, Blaser K, Akdis CA (2001) Histamine regulates T-cell and antibody responses by differential expression of H1 and H2 receptors. Nature 413:420–425

Jutel M, Watanabe T, Akdis M, Blaser K, Akdis CA (2002) Immune regulation by histamine. Curr Opin Immunol 14:735–740

Jutel M, Akdis M, Budak F, Aebischer-Casaulta C, Wrzyszcz M, Blaser K, Akdis CA (2003) IL-10 and TGF-beta cooperate in the regulatory T cell response to mucosal allergens in normal immunity and specific immunotherapy. Eur J Immunol 33:1205–1214

Jutel M, Jaeger L, Suck R, Meyer H, Fiebig H, Cromwell O (2005) Allergen-specific immunotherapy with recombinant grass pollen allergens. J Allergy Clin Immunol 116: 608–613

Kahler H, Stuwe H, Cromwell O, Fiebig H (1999) Reactivity of T cells with grass pollen allergen extract and allergoid. Int Arch Allergy Immunol 120:146–157

Kahlert H, Grage-Griebenow E, Stuwe HT, Cromwell O, Fiebig H (2000) T cell reactivity with allergoids: influence of the type of APC. J Immunol 165:1807–1815

Katz SI, Parker D, Turk JL (1974) B-cell suppression of delayed hypersensitivity reactions. Nature 251:550–551

Keskin O, Tuncer A, Adalioglu G, Sekerel BE, Sackesen C, Kalayci O (2006) The effects of grass pollen allergoid immunotherapy on clinical and immunological parameters in children with allergic rhinitis. Pediatr Allergy Immunol 17:396–407

Khattri R, Kasprowicz D, Cox T, Mortrud M, Appleby MW, Brunkow ME, Ziegler SF, Ramsdell F (2001) The amount of scurfin protein determines peripheral T cell number and responsiveness. J Immunol 167:6312–6320

Kiechl-Kohlendorfer U, Horak E, Mueller W, Strobl R, Haberland C, Fink FM, Schwaiger M, Gutenberger KH, Reich H, Meraner D, Kiechl S (2007) Neonatal characteristics and risk of atopic asthma in schoolchildren: results from a large prospective birth-cohort study. Acta Paediatr 96:1606–1610

Kraal G, Samsom JN, Mebius RE (2006) The importance of regional lymph nodes for mucosal tolerance. Immunol Rev 213:119–130

Kunzmann S, Mantel PY, Wohlfahrt JG, Akdis M, Blaser K, Schmidt-Weber CB (2003) Histamine enhances TGF-beta1-mediated suppression of Th2 responses. Faseb J 17: 1089–1095

La Grutta S, Arena A, D'Anneo WR, Gammeri E, Leonardi S, Trimarchi A, Platania D, La Rosa M (2007) Evaluation of the antiinflammatory and clinical effects of sublingual immunotherapy with carbamylated allergoid in allergic asthma with or without rhinitis. A 12-month perspective randomized, controlled, trial. Eur Ann Allergy Clin Immunol 39:40–44

Laffer S, Spitzauer S, Susani M, Pairleitner H, Schweiger C, Gronlund H, Menz G, Pauli G, Ishii T, Nolte H, Ebner C, Sehon AH, Kraft D, Eichler HG, Valenta R (1996) Comparison of recombinant timothy grass pollen allergens with natural extract for diagnosis of grass pollen allergy in different populations. J Allergy Clin Immunol 98:652–658

Larche M (2006) Immunoregulation by targeting T cells in the treatment of allergy and asthma. Curr Opin Immunol 18:745–750

Larche M (2007) Update on the current status of peptide immunotherapy. J Allergy Clin Immunol 119:906–909

Larenas-Linnemann D (2009) Sublingual immunotherapy in children: complete and updated review supporting evidence of effect. Curr Opin Allergy Clin Immunol 9:168–176

Letourneau S, Krieg C, Pantaleo G, Boyman O (2009) IL-2- and CD25-dependent immunoregulatory mechanisms in the homeostasis of T-cell subsets. J Allergy Clin Immunol 123:758–762

Leung DY, Bieber T (2003) Atopic dermatitis. Lancet 361:151–160

Lim S, Crawley E, Woo P, Barnes PJ (1998) Haplotype associated with low interleukin-10 production in patients with severe asthma. Lancet 352:113

Lim HW, Hillsamer P, Banham AH, Kim CH (2005) Cutting edge: direct suppression of B cells by CD4+CD25+ regulatory T cells. J Immunol 175:4180–4183

Ling EM, Smith T, Nguyen XD, Pridgeon C, Dallman M, Arbery J, Carr VA, Robinson DS (2004) Relation of CD4+CD25+ regulatory T-cell suppression of allergen-driven T-cell activation to atopic status and expression of allergic disease. Lancet 363:608–615

Lombardi V, Van Overtvelt L, Horiot S, Moussu H, Chabre H, Louise A, Balazuc AM, Mascarell L, Moingeon P (2008) Toll-like receptor 2 agonist Pam3CSK4 enhances the induction of antigen-specific tolerance via the sublingual route. Clin Exp Allergy 38:1819–1829

Lundy SK, Berlin AA, Lukacs NW (2003) Interleukin-12-independent down-modulation of cockroach antigen-induced asthma in mice by intranasal exposure to bacterial lipopolysaccharide. Am J Pathol 163:1961–1968

Manjarrez-Orduno N, Quach TD, Sanz I (2009) B cells and immunological tolerance. J Invest Dermatol 129:278–288

Marsh DG, Lichtenstein LM, Campbell DH (1970) Studies on "allergoids" prepared from naturally occurring allergens. I. Assay of allergenicity and antigenicity of formalinized rye group I component. Immunology 18:705–722

Matheson MC, Walters EH, Simpson JA, Wharton CL, Ponsonby AL, Johns DP, Jenkins MA, Giles GG, Hopper JL, Abramson MJ, Dharmage SC (2009) Relevance of the hygiene hypothesis to early vs. late onset allergic rhinitis. Clin Exp Allergy 39:370–378

Mazzoni A, Young HA, Spitzer JH, Visintin A, Segal DM (2001) Histamine regulates cytokine production in maturing dendritic cells, resulting in altered T cell polarization. J Clin Invest 108:1865–1873

McCaughtry TM, Hogquist KA (2008) Central tolerance: what have we learned from mice? Semin Immunopathol 30:399–409

McGee HS, Agrawal DK (2009) Naturally occurring and inducible T-regulatory cells modulating immune response in allergic asthma. Am J Respir Crit Care Med

Milovanovic M, Heine G, Zuberbier T, Worm M (2009) Allergen extract-induced interleukin-10 in human memory B cells inhibits immunoglobulin E production. Clin Exp Allergy 39: 671–678

Mistrello G, Brenna O, Roncarolo D, Zanoni D, Gentili M, Falagiani P (1996) Monomeric chemically modified allergens: immunologic and physicochemical characterization. Allergy 51:8–15

Mizoguchi A, Bhan AK (2006) A case for regulatory B cells. J Immunol 176:705–710

Mobs C, Slotosch C, Loffler H, Pfutzner W, Hertl M (2008) Cellular and humoral mechanisms of immune tolerance in immediate-type allergy induced by specific immunotherapy. Int Arch Allergy Immunol 147:171–178

Moingeon P, Batard T, Fadel R, Frati F, Sieber J, Van Overtvelt L (2006) Immune mechanisms of allergen-specific sublingual immunotherapy. Allergy 61:151–165

Moore KW, de Waal Malefyt R, Coffman RL, O'Garra A (2001) Interleukin-10 and the interleukin-10 receptor. Annu Rev Immunol 19:683–765

Moverare R, Elfman L, Vesterinen E, Metso T, Haahtela T (2002) Development of new IgE specificities to allergenic components in birch pollen extract during specific immunotherapy studied with immunoblotting and Pharmacia CAP System. Allergy 57:423–430

Neta R, Salvin SB (1974) Specific suppression of delayed hypersensitivity: the possible presence of a suppressor B cell in the regulation of delayed hypersensitivity. J Immunol 113:1716–1725

Nieminen K, Valovirta E, Savolainen J (2009) Clinical outcome and IL-17, IL-23, IL-27 and FOXP3 expression in peripheral blood mononuclear cells of pollen-allergic children during sublingual immunotherapy. Pediatr Allergy Immunol 21:e174–e84

Noon L (1955) Prophylactic inoculation against hay fever (historical document). Ann Allergy 13:713–716 passim

Nouri-Aria KT, Wachholz PA, Francis JN, Jacobson MR, Walker SM, Wilcock LK, Staple SQ, Aalberse RC, Till SJ, Durham SR (2004) Grass pollen immunotherapy induces mucosal and peripheral IL-10 responses and blocking IgG activity. J Immunol 172:3252–3259

Novak N, Bieber T, Leung DY (2003) Immune mechanisms leading to atopic dermatitis. J Allergy Clin Immunol 112:S128–S139

Ogawa Y, Duru EA, Ameredes BT (2008) Role of IL-10 in the resolution of airway inflammation. Curr Mol Med 8:437–445

Onishi Y, Fehervari Z, Yamaguchi T, Sakaguchi S (2008) Foxp3+ natural regulatory T cells preferentially form aggregates on dendritic cells in vitro and actively inhibit their maturation. Proc Natl Acad Sci USA 105:10113–10118

Osna N, Elliott K, Khan MM (2001) Regulation of interleukin-10 secretion by histamine in TH2 cells and splenocytes. Int Immunopharmacol 1:85–96

Ozdemir C, Akdis M, Akdis CA (2009) T regulatory cells and their counterparts: masters of immune regulation. Clin Exp Allergy 39:626–639

Palma-Carlos AG, Santos AS, Branco-Ferreira M, Pregal AL, Palma-Carlos ML, Bruno ME, Falagiani P, Riva G (2006) Clinical efficacy and safety of preseasonal sublingual

immunotherapy with grass pollen carbamylated allergoid in rhinitic patients. A double-blind, placebo-controlled study. Allergol Immunopathol (Madr) 34:194–198
Pauli G, Larsen TH, Rak S, Horak F, Pastorello E, Valenta R, Purohit A, Arvidsson M, Kavina A, Schroeder JW, Mothes N, Spitzauer S, Montagut A, Galvain S, Melac M, Andre C, Poulsen LK, Malling HJ (2008) Efficacy of recombinant birch pollen vaccine for the treatment of birch-allergic rhinoconjunctivitis. J Allergy Clin Immunol 122:951–960
Pelaia G, Renda T, Romeo P, Busceti MT, Maselli R (2008) Omalizumab in the treatment of severe asthma: efficacy and current problems. Ther Adv Respir Dis 2:409–421
Peng ZK, Naclerio RM, Norman PS, Adkinson NF Jr (1992) Quantitative IgE- and IgG-subclass responses during and after long-term ragweed immunotherapy. J Allergy Clin Immunol 89:519–529
Piccirillo CA, Shevach EM (2001) Cutting edge: control of CD8+ T cell activation by CD4+CD 25+ immunoregulatory cells. J Immunol 167:1137–1140
Pipet A, Botturi K, Pinot D, Vervloet D, Magnan A (2009) Allergen-specific immunotherapy in allergic rhinitis and asthma. Mechanisms and proof of efficacy. Respir Med 103:800–812
Pomes A (2008) Allergen structures and biologic functions: the cutting edge of allergy research. Curr Allergy Asthma Rep 8:425–432
Punnonen J, de Waal Malefyt R, van Vlasselaer P, Gauchat JF, de Vries JE (1993) IL-10 and viral IL-10 prevent IL-4-induced IgE synthesis by inhibiting the accessory cell function of monocytes. J Immunol 151:1280–1289
Radulovic S, Jacobson MR, Durham SR, Nouri-Aria KT (2008) Grass pollen immunotherapy induces Foxp3-expressi1472 e1461ng CD4+ CD25+ cells in the nasal mucosa. J Allergy Clin Immunol 121:1467–1472, 1472 e1461
Riedl MA (2008) The effect of air pollution on asthma and allergy. Curr Allergy Asthma Rep 8:139–146
Rossi RE, Monasterolo G, Coco G, Silvestro L, Operti D (2007) Evaluation of serum IgG4 antibodies specific to grass pollen allergen components in the follow up of allergic patients undergoing subcutaneous and sublingual immunotherapy. Vaccine 25:957–964
Satoguina JS, Weyand E, Larbi J, Hoerauf A (2005) T regulatory-1 cells induce IgG4 production by B cells: role of IL-10. J Immunol 174:4718–4726
Schandene L, Alonso-Vega C, Willems F, Gerard C, Delvaux A, Velu T, Devos R, de Boer M, Goldman M (1994) B7/CD28-dependent IL-5 production by human resting T cells is inhibited by IL-10. J Immunol 152:4368–4374
Schmidt-Weber CB, Blaser K (2005) New insights into the mechanisms of allergen-specific immunotherapy. Curr Opin Allergy Clin Immunol 5:525–530
Schmidt-Weber CB, Akdis M, Akdis CA (2007) TH17 cells in the big picture of immunology. J Allergy Clin Immunol 120:247–254
Seiskari T, Kondrashova A, Viskari H, Kaila M, Haapala AM, Aittoniemi J, Virta M, Hurme M, Uibo R, Knip M, Hyoty H (2007) Allergic sensitization and microbial load–a comparison between Finland and Russian Karelia. Clin Exp Immunol 148:47–52
Sicherer SH, Leung DY (2009) Advances in allergic skin disease, anaphylaxis, and hypersensitivity reactions to foods, drugs, and insects in 2008. J Allergy Clin Immunol 123:319–327
Singh A, Carson WF IV, Secor ER Jr, Guernsey LA, Flavell RA, Clark RB, Thrall RS, Schramm CM (2008) Regulatory role of B cells in a murine model of allergic airway disease. J Immunol 180:7318–7326
Srivastava D, Arora N, Singh BP (2009) Current immunological approaches for management of allergic rhinitis and bronchial asthma. Inflamm Res 58:523–536
Strachan DP (1989) Hay fever, hygiene, and household size. BMJ 299:1259–1260
Strachan DP (2000) Family size, infection and atopy: the first decade of the "hygiene hypothesis". Thorax 55(Suppl 1):S2–S10
Strait RT, Morris SC, Finkelman FD (2006) IgG-blocking antibodies inhibit IgE-mediated anaphylaxis in vivo through both antigen interception and Fc gamma RIIb cross-linking. J Clin Invest 116:833–841

Sun JB, Cuburu N, Blomquist M, Li BL, Czerkinsky C, Holmgren J (2006) Sublingual tolerance induction with antigen conjugated to cholera toxin B subunit induces Foxp3+CD25+CD4+ regulatory T cells and suppresses delayed-type hypersensitivity reactions. Scand J Immunol 64:251–259

Sun JB, Flach CF, Czerkinsky C, Holmgren J (2008) B lymphocytes promote expansion of regulatory T cells in oral tolerance: powerful induction by antigen coupled to cholera toxin B subunit. J Immunol 181:8278–8287

Szalai K, Jensen-Jarolim E, Pali-Scholl I (2008) Vaccination strategies based on the mimotope concept. G Ital Dermatol Venereol 143:95–104

Tauro S, Su YC, Thomas S, Schwarze J, Matthaei KI, Townsend D, Simson L, Tripp RA, Mahalingam S (2008) Molecular and cellular mechanisms in the viral exacerbation of asthma. Microbes Infect 10:1014–1023

Trivedi B, Valerio C, Slater JE (2003) Endotoxin content of standardized allergen vaccines. J Allergy Clin Immunol 111:777–783

Tsitoura DC, Yeung VP, DeKruyff RH, Umetsu DT (2002) Critical role of B cells in the development of T cell tolerance to aeroallergens. Int Immunol 14:659–667

Valenta R, Vrtala S, Laffer S, Spitzauer S, Kraft D (1998) Recombinant allergens. Allergy 53: 552–561

Van Bruaene N, Perez-Novo CA, Basinski TM, Van Zele T, Holtappels G, De Ruyck N, Schmidt-Weber C, Akdis C, Van Cauwenberge P, Bachert C, Gevaert P (2008) T-cell regulation in chronic paranasal sinus disease. J Allergy Clin Immunol 121:1435–1441, 1441 e1431–1433

van der Veen MJ, Mulder M, Witteman AM, van Ree R, Aalberse RC, Jansen HM, van der Zee JS (1996) False-positive skin prick test responses to commercially available dog dander extracts caused by contamination with house dust mite (Dermatophagoides pteronyssinus) allergens. J Allergy Clin Immunol 98:1028–1034

van Hage-Hamsten M, Kronqvist M, Zetterstrom O, Johansson E, Niederberger V, Vrtala S, Gronlund H, Gronneberg R, Valenta R (1999) Skin test evaluation of genetically engineered hypoallergenic derivatives of the major birch pollen allergen, Bet v 1: results obtained with a mix of two recombinant Bet v 1 fragments and recombinant Bet v 1 trimer in a Swedish population before the birch pollen season. J Allergy Clin Immunol 104:969–977

van Helvoort JM, Samsom JN, Chantry D, Jansen W, Schadee-Eestermans I, Thepen T, Mebius RE, Kraal G (2004) Preferential expression of IgG2b in nose draining cervical lymph nodes and its putative role in mucosal tolerance induction. Allergy 59:1211–1218

van Neerven RJ, Wikborg T, Lund G, Jacobsen B, Brinch-Nielsen A, Arnved J, Ipsen H (1999) Blocking antibodies induced by specific allergy vaccination prevent the activation of CD4 + T cells by inhibiting serum-IgE-facilitated allergen presentation. J Immunol 163:2944–2952

Van Ree R, Van Leeuwen WA, Dieges PH, Van Wijk RG, De Jong N, Brewczyski PZ, Kroon AM, Schilte PP, Tan KY, Simon-Licht IF, Roberts AM, Stapel SO, Aalberse RC (1997) Measurement of IgE antibodies against purified grass pollen allergens (Lol p 1, 2, 3 and 5) during immunotherapy. Clin Exp Allergy 27:68–74

van Wijk RG (2008) When to initiate immunotherapy in children with allergic disease? Lessons from the paediatric studies. Curr Opin Allergy Clin Immunol 8:565–570

Veldhoen M, Uyttenhove C, van Snick J, Helmby H, Westendorf A, Buer J, Martin B, Wilhelm C, Stockinger B (2008) Transforming growth factor-beta 'reprograms' the differentiation of T helper 2 cells and promotes an interleukin 9-producing subset. Nat Immunol 9:1341–1346

Velickovic TC, Jankov RM (2008) Design and modifications of allergens for improving specific immunotherapy. Inflamm Allergy Drug Targets 7:270–278

Verhoef A, Alexander C, Kay AB, Larche M (2005) T cell epitope immunotherapy induces a CD4+ T cell population with regulatory activity. PLoS Med 2:e78

von Mutius E, Radon K (2008) Living on a farm: impact on asthma induction and clinical course. Immunol Allergy Clin North Am 28:631–647, ix-x

Vrtala S (2008) From allergen genes to new forms of allergy diagnosis and treatment. Allergy 63:299–309

Vrtala S, Sperr WR, Reimitzer I, van Ree R, Laffer S, Muller WD, Valent P, Lechner K, Rumpold H, Kraft D et al (1993) cDNA cloning of a major allergen from timothy grass (Phleum pratense) pollen; characterization of the recombinant Phl pV allergen. J Immunol 151: 4773–4781

Vrtala S, Hirtenlehner K, Susani M, Hufnagl P, Binder BR, Vangelista L, Pastore A, Sperr WR, Valent P, Ebner C, Kraft D, Valenta R (1999) Genetic engineering of recombinant hypoallergenic oligomers of the major birch pollen allergen, Bet v 1: candidates for specific immunotherapy. Int Arch Allergy Immunol 118:218–219

Vrtala S, Akdis CA, Budak F, Akdis M, Blaser K, Kraft D, Valenta R (2000) T cell epitope-containing hypoallergenic recombinant fragments of the major birch pollen allergen, Bet v 1, induce blocking antibodies. J Immunol 165:6653–6659

Wachholz PA, Soni NK, Till SJ, Durham SR (2003) Inhibition of allergen-IgE binding to B cells by IgG antibodies after grass pollen immunotherapy. J Allergy Clin Immunol 112:915–922

Wagner S, Radauer C, Bublin M, Hoffmann-Sommergruber K, Kopp T, Greisenegger EK, Vogel L, Vieths S, Scheiner O, Breiteneder H (2008) Naturally occurring hypoallergenic Bet v 1 isoforms fail to induce IgE responses in individuals with birch pollen allergy. J Allergy Clin Immunol 121:246–252

Walgraffe D, Matteotti C, El Bakkoury M, Garcia L, Marchand C, Bullens D, Vandenbranden M, Jacquet A (2009) A hypoallergenic variant of Der p 1 as a candidate for mite allergy vaccines. J Allergy Clin Immunol 123:1150–1156

Walters S, Webster KE, Sutherland A, Gardam S, Groom J, Liuwantara D, Marino E, Thaxton J, Weinberg A, Mackay F, Brink R, Sprent J, Grey ST (2009) Increased CD4+Foxp3+ T cells in BAFF-transgenic mice suppress T cell effector responses. J Immunol 182:793–801

Waterhouse P, Penninger JM, Timms E, Wakeham A, Shahinian A, Lee KP, Thompson CB, Griesser H, Mak TW (1995) Lymphoproliferative disorders with early lethality in mice deficient in Ctla-4. Science 270:985–988

Wells AD (2009) New insights into the molecular basis of T cell anergy: anergy factors, avoidance sensors, and epigenetic imprinting. J Immunol 182:7331–7341

Werfel T, Morita A, Grewe M, Renz H, Wahn U, Krutmann J, Kapp A (1996) Allergen specificity of skin-infiltrating T cells is not restricted to a type-2 cytokine pattern in chronic skin lesions of atopic dermatitis. J Invest Dermatol 107:871–876

Williams A, Henzgen M, Rajakulasingam K (2007) Additional benefit of a third year of specific grass pollen allergoid immunotherapy in patients with seasonal allergic rhinitis. Eur Ann Allergy Clin Immunol 39:123–126

Wilson DR, Lima MT, Durham SR (2005) Sublingual immunotherapy for allergic rhinitis: systematic review and meta-analysis. Allergy 60:4–12

Wing K, Onishi Y, Prieto-Martin P, Yamaguchi T, Miyara M, Fehervari Z, Nomura T, Sakaguchi S (2008) CTLA-4 control over Foxp3+ regulatory T cell function. Science 322:271–275

Workman CJ, Szymczak-Workman AL, Collison LW, Pillai MR, Vignali DA (2009) The development and function of regulatory T cells. Cell Mol Life Sci

Yamazaki S, Steinman RM (2009) Dendritic cells as controllers of antigen-specific Foxp3+ regulatory T cells. J Dermatol Sci 54:69–75

Yazi D, Akkoc T, Ozdemir C, Yesil O, Aydogan M, Sancak R, Bahceciler NN, Barlan IB (2007) Long-term modulatory effect of Mycobacterium vaccae treatment on histopathologic changes in a murine model of asthma. Ann Allergy Asthma Immunol 98:573–579

Zakzuk J, Jimenez S, Cheong N, Puerta L, Lee BW, Chua KY, Caraballo L (2009) Immunological characterization of a Blo t 12 isoallergen: identification of immunoglobulin E epitopes. Clin Exp Allergy 39:608–616

Zuany-Amorim C, Haile S, Leduc D, Dumarey C, Huerre M, Vargaftig BB, Pretolani M (1995) Interleukin-10 inhibits antigen-induced cellular recruitment into the airways of sensitized mice. J Clin Invest 95:2644–2651

Clinical Experience with Recombinant Molecules for Allergy Vaccination

Oliver Cromwell, Verena Niederberger, Friedrich Horak and Helmut Fiebig

Abstract Numerous allergens have been cloned and produced by the use of recombinant DNA technology. In several cases recombinant variants with reduced IgE-reactivity have also been developed as candidates for allergen specific immunotherapy. Only very few of these proteins have as yet been tested in the clinic, and the major focus has been on birch and grass pollen, two of the most common causes of IgE-mediated allergic disease. This article serves to justify the rational for using recombinant products and reviews the progress that has been made to date with their clinical assessment.

Contents

O. Cromwell (✉) · H. Fiebig
Allergopharma Joachim Ganzer KG, Hermann-Koerner-Strasse 52,
21465 Reinbek, Germany
e-mail: oliver.cromwell@allergopharma.de

V. Niederberger
Department of Otorhinolaryngology, Medical University of Vienna,
Vienna, Austria

F. Horak
ENT University Clinic, University of Vienna,
Vienna, Austria

Current Topics in Microbiology and Immunology (2011) 352: 27–42
DOI: 10.1007/82_2011_129

Published Online: 12 May 2011

The first publication describing the use of recombinant DNA technology to clone and express an allergen appeared in 1988 (Breiteneder et al. 1988, 1989) and since that time several hundred other allergens have been produced in recombinant form and characterized (Allergome 2009). There have also been numerous reports on the development of recombinant allergen variants with reduced IgE-reactivity as candidates for specific immunotherapy (Ferreira et al. 2006; Niederberger and Valenta 2006). The only substantial clinical studies conducted to date have been with recombinant allergens or allergen derivatives of grass and birch pollen, two of the most common causes of IgE-mediated allergic disease. Recombinant house dust mite and cat allergens have also been the focus of extensive preclinical development work. A small clinical study using recombinant Fel d 1 has already been reported and it seems likely that the group 1 and 2 allergens of house dust mites will soon be the subject of clinical trials. Before such products can be granted marketing licenses and placed on the market it will be necessary to demonstrate their clinical efficacy and safety. This article serves to justify the rationale for using recombinant products and review the progress that has been made to date with their clinical assessment.

1 Considerations for Optimal Allergen Specific Immunotherapy

Allergen specific immunotherapy is a causal treatment for IgE-mediated allergic disease, in other words the allergen responsible for sensitization and provoking symptoms of rhinoconjunctivitis, allergic asthma etc. is administered under controlled conditions in order to change the course of the immune response and thereby ameliorate symptoms. Characterization of the cytokine profiles of allergen specific human T cells revealed that the immune responses of healthy and allergic subjects to common environmental allergens can be defined in terms of a delicate balance between allergen specific T helper type 2 (Th2) and inducible type 1 T regulatory (Tr1) cells (Akdis et al. 2004). The Th2 cells of the allergic phenotype are associated with interleukin (IL)-4, IL-5 and IL-13, which promote IgE production and allergic inflammation, while Tr1 cells are particularly linked with the cytokine IL-10. Tr1 and Th3 regulatory cell phenotypes that secrete the suppressive cytokines IL-10 and TGF-β, respectively have been associated with induction of peripheral T cell tolerance in allergic subjects undergoing successful immunotherapy with bee venom and aeroallergens (Akdis et al. 1998; Jutel et al. 2003). whilst low allergen doses favor a Th2 cytokine response and a switch to IgE, high allergen doses favor induction of regulatory T cells and an enhanced Th1 cytokine profile together with modification or down-regulation of the Th2 phenotype (Larche et al. 2006). This is consistent with the data from studies in bee-keepers subjected to repeated bee stings which showed that high dose allergen tolerance is associated with clonal expansion of allergen specific IL-10-producing Tr1 cells.

Investigations with bee venom phospholipase (PLA) specific T cell clones from subjects either allergic, hyposensitized or immune (protected) to bee stings have shown that both absolute and relative amounts of secreted cytokines depend on the antigen concentration. Low antigen doses induced IL-4 production, but little or no IFN-γ, whereas significant amounts of both cytokines were obtained at higher PLA concentrations. T-cell clones from allergic and hyposensitized individuals required higher critical amounts of antigen for IFN-γ induction, and expressed increasing IL-4/IFN-γ ratios with increasing concentrations of PLA (Carballido et al. 1992). Therefore modulation of cytokine patterns is dependent on the dose of antigen, and high dose is important for induction of a protective immune response. These conclusions are supported by studies in mice (Ruedl et al. 2000) as well as by results for allergen specific immunotherapy in man which clearly show that a higher dose is more clinically effective (Frew et al. 2006).

Allergen specific immunotherapy is conducted using extracts of natural raw materials containing the appropriate allergens together with numerous other proteins and molecules from the plant or animal material in question. The concentrations of the allergens are dictated to a large extent by the raw material, and while some allergens may be well represented others may only be present in concentrations that are not sufficient to achieve an optimal clinical benefit. The use of allergens or allergen variants derived through the use of recombinant DNA technology provides an opportunity to create products which include only the relevant allergens in concentrations suitable for achieving optimal clinical benefit. The concentrations of all components can be declared in mass units and it will be possible to achieve excellent product consistency.

Allergen concentration is also relevant with regard to the possibility of inducing new sensitizations. Provided that the allergens or allergen derivatives are present in sufficiently high concentrations in a preparation administered for subcutaneous specific immunotherapy which by-passes the mucosa, it is unlikely that they will favor IgE production, but rather induction of peripheral T cell tolerance. By way of example, birch pollen allergic subjects who were sensitized predominantly to Bet v 1 and underwent treatment with a birch pollen extract developed new sensitivities to what are normally considered as minor birch pollen allergens that are not present in anything like the same concentration as Bet v 1(Moverare et al. 2002). It is not yet clear if similar considerations apply for sublingual immunotherapy which has a clear booster effect on existing IgE responses (Didier et al. 2007; Dahl et al. 2008) and may well involve other mechanisms of action. These are areas that are worthy of further investigation.

It will not be realistic to produce every protein component of an allergen extract using recombinant DNA technology for inclusion in a therapeutic preparation. Therefore the first objective of a clinical development program has to be the identification of an adequate combination of proteins to achieve a clinically relevant benefit for the patients. In the case of birch pollen and cat allergy it appears that Bet v 1 and Fel d 1, respectively are sufficient, but in the cases of grass pollen and house dust mite allergy two or more allergens will be essential. It is important to establish these basic requirements before going ahead with studies with hypoallergenic variants, since in the case of an unsuccessful study it would be difficult to decide if the result was attributable to the lack of an important allergen or an ineffective variant.

2 Allergen Variants with Reduced IgE-Binding Activity

One of the potential risks of this causal treatment is that it may induce allergen associated side effects, and at worst life-threatening anaphylactic reactions. This consideration was one factor that prompted the development of hypoallergenic derivatives produced by chemical modification of the allergen extracts (Maasch and Marsh 1987). Such preparations are intended to minimize the risk of inducing IgE-mediated reactions, while ensuring the possibility for administering an adequately high dose to favor a therapeutic effect. The reduced IgE-reactivity minimizes the potential to activate mast cells and basophils with the release of inflammatory mediators. Furthermore, IgE antibody-dependent uptake by antigen presenting cells, which would normally favor promotion of the allergic phenotype with production of Th2 cytokines and allergen specific IgE (van der Heijden et al. 1993), is also excluded (Akdis and Blaser 2001). Chemically modified allergen extracts (allergoids) have found widespread acceptance. The choice of chemical method used to produce the allergoids determines which types of chemical residues in the proteins will be subject to modification, but it is not possible to target specific sites within a protein. The advent of recombinant DNA technology provides the opportunity to use genetic engineering techniques to develop tailor-made hypoallergenic molecules which may present some additional advantages for allergen specific immunotherapy. Not only is it possible to compromise the IgE-reactivity of the proteins, but there is also the possibility to enhance the immunogenicity and introduce features that can influence the processing of an allergen by the immune system.

The design features of engineered hypoallergenic variants can be precisely defined and validated with respect to the intended specific immunotherapeutic application. Genetic detoxification of bacterial toxins by gene mutations at sites coding for the amino acids involved in the enzymatic sites, and thus the toxic effects, has already been achieved (Rappuoli et al. 1995), thus providing an alternative to the toxoids produced by chemical modification. In such cases the choice of mutation site is relatively straight-forward, but this is often not the case with allergens in which the IgE-binding epitopes rely principally on the conformation of the protein. Several strategies have been adopted in order to impart hypoallergenic characteristics to allergens without compromising T-cell reactivity and immunomodulatory potential, and experience has shown that such strategies have to be tailored to match the characteristics of each individual allergen. A bigger challenge is often presented by the search for a molecular variant that can be expressed and recovered in a soluble form in adequate amounts with consistent characteristics and quality.

It is important to define the criteria which a hypoallergenic variant has to fulfill before the decision can be made to take it into clinical testing. A variant must have advantages for a very large majority of potential recipients, that is to say it must have obvious hypoallergenic characteristics for all those patients. Allergic subjects differ widely in terms of the amounts of specific IgE antibody they produce against a particular allergen, and furthermore the spectrum and the number of epitopes recognized may vary. Consequently it is not sufficient to compromise reactivity of only one of several IgE-binding epitopes in an allergen, and it is important to screen new variants with a library of sera from allergic subjects in order to cover all IgE-binding epitopes. It is usually not appropriate to use pool sera to assess hypoallergenic characteristics. If only a small number of sera in the pool react strongly with a variant their contribution would be diluted by a large number of weak reactors. Furthermore various different methods should be used to assess the derivatives, including solid-phase and liquid-phase immunoassays and cellular assays such as basophil activation or histamine release. Skin or provocation testing may then be used to confirm hypoallergenic characteristics in vivo. Ideally hypoallergenic characteristics should be observed consistently with all test methods. Finally, the reduction in IgE-reactivity should be sufficient to confer a meaningful advantage.

3 Recombinant Grass and Birch Pollen Allergens

The grass *Phleum pratense* is a member of the sub-family *Pooideae*, which in turn belongs to the family *Poaceae*. It shows very substantial cross-reactivity with other members of the sub-family (Andersson and Lidholm 2003; Johansen et al. 2009) and can therefore be considered as representative of grasses found in temperate regions. The allergens Phl p 1, Phl p 2, Phl p 5a, Phl p 5b and Phl p 6 account for a substantial proportion of the specific IgE sensitization developed against grass pollen. Recombinant forms of these five allergens were the basis of a preparation investigated in a double blind placebo controlled clinical trial in 62 grass pollen allergic patients suffering from rhinoconjunctivitis with or without asthma (Jutel et al. 2005). Aluminium hydroxide adsorbates of the individual recombinant allergens were used as a mixture and administered by subcutaneous injection with increasing concentrations at 7-day intervals prior to the grass pollen season, starting with 0.02 μg total protein, followed by 0.16 μg and then doubling to 40 μg total protein (0.8 ml). The maximum dose contained 10 μg Phlp1, 5μg Phlp2, 10 μg Phlp5a, 10 μg Phlp5b and 5 μg Phlp6. Maintenance injections were then continued until after the subsequent pollen season, with a 50% reduction during each pollen season, so that the total period of treatment was 18 months.

The primary outcome measure to assess clinical efficacy was a combined symptom-medication score (SMS) derived from patients' diaries. Diaries were kept for 3 month periods encompassing each pollen season, and provided a record of the nature and severity of eye, nose and chest symptoms, together with the type and dose of any rescue medication. A preprotocol analysis included 24 active treatment and 25 placebo patients, and showed a 39% improvement in the active treatment group relative to placebo ($p = 0.041$). Symptoms alone improved by 37% ($p = 0.015$) and the use of symptomatic medication decreased by 36.5% relative to placebo. The preparation showed a favorable safety profile.

A validated rhinitis quality of life questionnaire (RQLQ) (Juniper and Guyatt 1991) registered benefits for those subjects on active treatment by comparison with placebo during the first pollen season, and these increased still further during the second pollen season with an overall significant benefit ($p = 0.024$), providing further evidence of clinical efficacy. Significant effects were registered in 5 of 7 domains tested, with the mean differences between active and placebo treatment substantially in excess of a score of 0.5 that may be considered as a level of clinical relevance. Active treatment also increased allergen tolerance as judged in a conjunctival provocation test with a standardized 6-grass allergen extract. The effect failed to achieve statistical significance, very probably as a consequence of the relatively small number of patients. Taken together the results indicate that the mixture of five allergens is sufficient to achieve good clinical benefit.

Those subjects treated with the recombinant allergen preparation showed large and highly significant increases in both IgG1 and IgG4 allergen specific antibody concentrations together with a significant decrease in specific IgE. The specific IgG1 concentration increased approximately 60-fold, peaking during the first 12 months of the study. IgG4 showed a continuing upward trend, achieving an approximately 4000-fold increase by the end of the 18 month treatment period. Specific IgE levels were not significantly different between groups at the beginning of the study, but thereafter the active treatment group showed a downward trend with values significantly less than baseline. Phl p 5a/b specific IgE antibodies were not detected in four subjects from each group prior to the treatment, although all reacted to Phl p 1 and other grass pollen allergens. None of these subjects developed Phl p 5a/b reactive IgE antibodies during the study, although the 4 subjects receiving active treatment developed strong IgG4 and IgG1 Phl p 5a/b responses indicative of either pre-existing immunity to the allergen without class-switching to IgE or induction of immunity.This observation needs to be substantiated and is relevant to the possible prophylactic effects of specific immunotherapy and guarding against the development of new sensitizations.

The same five grass pollen allergens in the same relative concentrations were formulated with total protein concentrations of 20, 40, 80 or 120 μg per maximum dose and used in a randomized, double blind, placebo controlled dose finding study with 10 subjects per group. Grass pollen allergic patients were treated for approximately 3 months prior to the grass pollen season. Primary endpoint in this study was the number of grade III and IV systemic reactions graded according to Tryba (1994), and the main secondary endpoints the early and late phase reactions in intracutaneous tests. Despite the fact that the 120μg dose contained 30μg of each of Phl p 1, Phl p 5a and Phl p 5b, some of the highest concentrations tested to date for subcutaneous immunotherapy, safety was very good and there were no drop-outs attributable to side effects. The use of progressive dosage increases probably contributes to this good safety record.

The early and late phase responses after a titrated intra-cutaneous test were able to discriminate between the different therapeutic dosage schedules with decreases in the magnitude of the skin reactions with increasing therapeutic dose (Sprung et al. 2009). Grass pollen specific IgG1 and IgG4 antibody responses were seen in all active treatment groups, but not in the placebo group. The *Phleum* preparation has now entered Phase III clinical testing.

One question that frequently arises is - how do the results with a recombinant allergen compare with those for a natural allergen? A study in birch pollen allergic subjects addressed this by comparing natural and recombinant Bet v 1 with placebo, and went one step further by including a group of subjects treated with a whole birch pollen preparation (Pauli et al. 2008). Treatment commenced 6 months prior to the expected peak of the birch pollen season, and the Bet v 1 major allergen dose was increased progressively from 0.05 to a maximum of 15.0 μg at weekly intervals. Treatment was extended over 2 years with monthly injections of the maximum dose. Significant reductions in rhinoconjunctivitis symptoms were seen after one year of treatment and these were increased still further to circa 50% in each of the three active treatment groups by comparison with placebo. The use of rescue medication was significantly reduced by the order of 65% in all active treatment groups. Skin test sensitivity also decreased significantly in all three active treatment groups, and interestingly the reduction in the group treated with recombinant Bet v 1 was significantly larger than those in the birch pollen and natural Bet v 1 groups. Marked increases in Bet v 1 specific IgG were seen in each of the treatment groups. No new IgE sensitizations were observed in the recombinant and natural Bet v 1 groups, but sensitivities to Bet v 2 were induced in 3/29 subjects treated with the pollen preparation.

4 Recombinant Hypoallergenic Variants of Birch Pollen Allergen Bet v 1

The IgE-binding reactivity of allergens such as Bet v 1 from birch pollen is very dependent on their 3-D structure. Cleaving the cDNA and expressing the two parts separately results in two allergen fragments (amino acid residues 1–73 and 74–159) showing random coil conformation (Vrtala et al. 1997). This loss of conformation almost certainly accounts for the loss of IgE-antibody binding activity. The cleavage point was chosen so as not to compromise recognized T cell epitopes (Vrtala et al. 2001a).

The birch pollen protein has also been used as a model system to investigate the potential of oligomerization to influence IgE-reactivity. Linking three copies of the Bet v 1 cDNA in sequence and expression in *E. coli* resulted in a trimeric form of the protein. IgE-reactivity was reduced, as judged by histamine release and skin testing, but circular dichroism spectroscopy showed that secondary structure was essentially the same as monomeric Bet v 1 (Vrtala et al. 2001b). Basophil activation measured in terms of CD203c expression indicated that the trimer is hypoallergenic, but less so than the fragments (Kahlert et al. 2003). Steric hindrance of the IgE-binding sites is the probable explanation for the hypoallergenic characteristics.

Skin prick tests with concentrations of 100 μg/ml of the fragments or the trimer in subjects with a positive response to native Bet v 1 showed that 18 of 23 and 15 of 23 subjects failed to react to the fragment mixture and the trimer, respectively (van Hage-Hamsten et al. 1999). A similar result emerged from intradermal testing, with 8 of 23 and 13 of 23 of the birch pollen allergic subjects failing to react to 1 μg/ml concentrations of the fragment mixture and the trimer, respectively. Clear dose response effects were seen with each of the allergen derivatives. The Bet v 1 fragments were tested separately and both were shown to be hypoallergenic in nature. A second study produced very similar results (Pauli et al. 2000). However it was observed that there was a very large inter-subject variation in the end-point of the intradermal tests, although both derivatives showed hypoallergenic characteristics to one degree or another. It is important to realize that such preparations are only going to offer advantages for safety and higher dosing if those advantages apply for all patients.

The first study of allergen specific immunotherapy with recombinant preparations investigated the clinical effects, immunological activity and tolerance of a mixture of the two Bet v 1 fragments and the Bet v 1 trimer in comparison to placebo. The recombinant preparations were adsorbed to aluminium hydroxide suspensions at concentrations of 100 μg/ml, and immunotherapy was conducted with a course of 8 pre-seasonal injections of increasing concentrations from 1 to 80 μg total protein, with further injections of the maximum concentration up until the beginning of the pollen season (Niederberger et al. 2004; Purohit et al. 2008). The results of the study were confounded to some extent by very different pollen counts in the three study centers and substantial counts of cross-reactive alder pollen several weeks in advance of the birch pollen season in one of the centers.

A combined symptom-medication score and a visual analogue score failed to reveal any significant differences between active and placebo treatments. Within-group comparisons, excluding those subjects from the center without a substantial pollen count, showed a significant improvement for the trimer group. Significant decreases in nasal sensitivity to allergen were seen in the fragment and trimer groups, but they did not differ significantly from placebo. All three study groups showed decreased skin test sensitivity. Local injection site reactions were most frequent in the trimer group and occurred soon after injection, whereas those in the fragment group generally occurred after several hours. Systemic reactions were elicited more frequently by fragments. These results together with the variations in hypoallergenic characteristics between birch pollen allergic subjects contributed to a decision not to pursue the clinical development of these preparations.

Withstanding the disappointing clinical data, both the fragment and trimer preparations of Bet v 1 proved to be strong immunogens inducing Bet v 1 specific

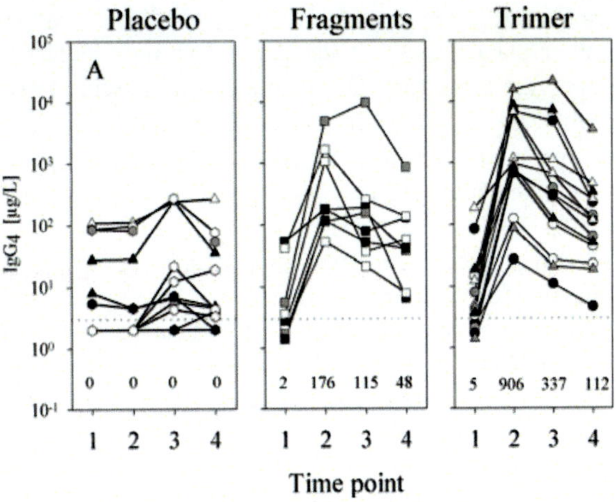

Fig. 1 Bet v 1 specific IgG4 antibody responses during the course of specific immunotherapy with a Bet v 1 trimer (n = 14), Bet v 1 fragments (n = 8) and placebo (n = 20). Data from one of three study centers (Vienna) for blood samples collected 1: before pre-seasonal immunotherapy; 2: after immunotherapy; 3: after the birch pollen season; and 4: 12 months after the first sample. (Purohit et al. 2008)

IgG1 and IgG4 antibody responses that peaked at the end of treatment with concentrations in the order of 100-fold more than those at baseline (Fig. 1). IgG2 and IgA antibody responses were also documented for subjects in both active treatment arms in one of the three study centers. Increases in Bet v 1 specific IgE during seasonal pollen exposure were blunted in the active treatment groups by comparison with placebo.

The serum antibodies were shown to be able to inhibit allergen induced histamine release in vitro from basophils of birch pollen allergic subjects (Niederberger et al. 2004). It was possible to show correlations between IgG1 antibody titers and both improvement in clinical symptoms, as judged by a ten-point interval scale, and reduction in skin test reactivity to Bet v 1.

Bet v 1 specific antibody responses were measured in nasal lavage fluids from a randomly selected sub-group of 23 subjects at the end of the birch pollen season following the course of immunotherapy and again 12 months after the time point at which treatment had commenced (Reisinger et al. 2005). Bet v 1 specific lavage fluid IgG1 levels were significantly raised at the end of the pollen season in those subjects that had received the active preparations (10 in trimer and 3 in fragment mixture groups) in comparison with placebo. Higher levels of IgG2 and IgG4 were also detected, as was the case in serum, but these were not significant. There were also no apparent differences in IgA levels. There were correlations between the various IgG subgroup concentrations in serum and lavage fluid. At the end of the birch pollen season there was a correlation between nasal IgG4 and reduced specific nasal sensitivity. Perhaps not surprisingly, the nasal antibody levels mirrored those in serum. The reduced nasal sensitivity may be accounted for by the inhibitory effect of the antibodies on basophil and mast cell mediator release as was demonstrated for the serum antibodies in vitro.

The possibility that immunotherapy with the fragments and trimer might also provide benefit for patients with birch pollen associated oral allergy syndrome (OAS) was also considered. A sub-group of 44 patients from one study centre who suffered from symptoms of OAS attributable to apples, hazel nuts, carrot, celery or other plant derived foods showed various increases in IgG1 and IgG4 to major allergens from these foodstuffs (Niederberger et al. 2007). Antibody responses in other antibody classes appeared not to be affected. Seven of 25 actively treated subjects reported improvements in their OAS compared with only one from 19 in the placebo group. Two placebo and 2 actively treated subjects reported worsened OAS.

Investigations into cytokine responses showed that treatment with trimer resulted in significant reductions in IL-5 and IL-13 producing cells compared between pre- and post treatment, which was indicative of a suppression of the Th2 response (Gafvelin et al. 2005). There were also trends for decreased numbers of IL-4 producing cells and increased numbers of IL-12 producing cells, but differences were not significant, very probably because of the small subject numbers (8 in trimer, 10 in fragment mixture and 8 in placebo groups). The results from the various antibody and cytokine measurements provide an encouraging basis for pursuing the further development of hypoallergenic derivatives per se, but emphasis has to be placed on the generation of data to provide evidence of clinical efficacy.

An alternative strategy for developing a hypoallergenic derivative came from the observation that recombinant Bet v 1 can be induced to adopt a stable largely random coil structure which can be clearly distinguished from the secondary structure of the native molecule by circular dichroism spectroscopy. This folding variant, designated Bet v 1-FV, exhibits hypoallergenic properties as judged by immunoassay inhibition tests and basophil activation (Fig. 2) (Kahlert et al. 2008; Weber et al. 2003). An open, randomized comparative clinical study with recombinant Bet v 1-FV and a natural birch pollen extract was started in 2003 (Klimek et al. 2005; Narkus et al. 2009). Treatment with aluminium hydroxide adsorbed preparations of the allergens was administered to subjects with birch pollen rhinitis over a period of four months prior to the birch pollen season with injections at weekly intervals. The maximum dose of the hypoallergenic recombinant preparation was 80 μg, approximately four-fold higher than the Bet v 1 in the whole pollen preparation. The combined SMS for subjects receiving the recombinant preparation was favorably less than that for the subjects receiving the natural pollen extract, and the scores for both groups superior to those of a reference group with only anti-symptomatic treatment (parallel control group). A second course of preseasonal immunotherapy was administered prior to the next pollen season, and then both groups showed similar combined symptom/medication scores (Fig. 3) (Kettner et al. 2007a; Narkus et al. 2009). Improvements in specific nasal sensitivity, as judged by a nasal provocation test, were seen in both study groups, and the immunogenic activity of the preparations was confirmed by their ability to induce strong IgG1 and IgG4 antibody responses. Safety data indicated that the preparations were comparable with respect to the occurrence of adverse events. A subsequent double blind placebo controlled study in subjects with symptoms of rhinoconjunctivitis, and with more than 100 subjects in each arm, has confirmed the clinical efficacy of the recombinant preparation (Kettner et al. 2007b). Symptoms and use of rescue medication were documented

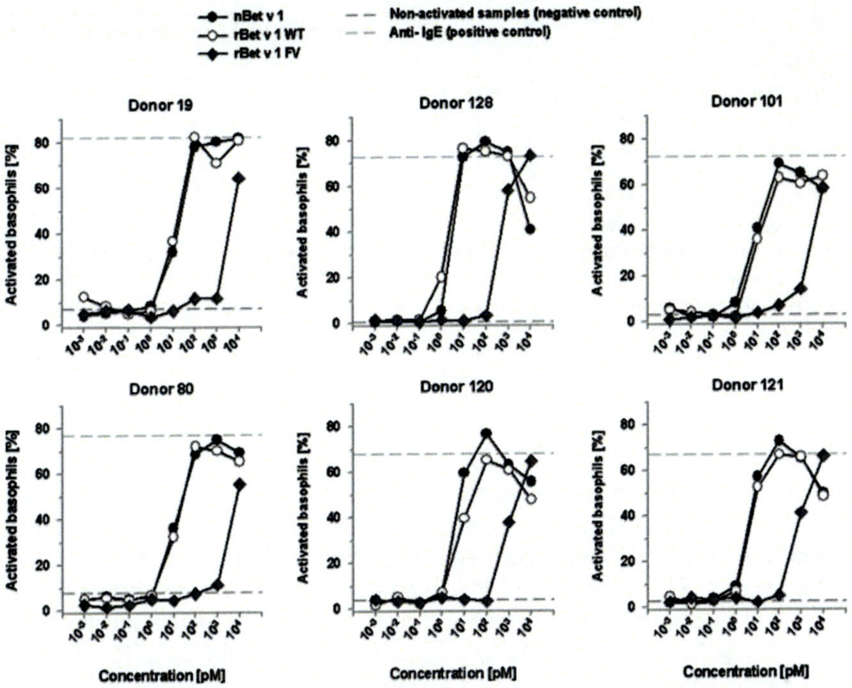

Fig. 2 Stimulation of basophils from whole blood with different concentrations of nBet v 1, rBet v 1-FV and rBet v 1-WT. Basophil activation was determined using CD203c expression. The proteins were tested in serial dilutions in a concentration range from 0.001 to 10,000 pM (Kahlert et al. 2008)

in a baseline year. Subjects received an 18 month course of immunotherapy starting four months prior to the expected pollen season such that they were established on a maximum maintenance dose of 80 μg prior to pollen exposure. Therapy was continued through out the end of the subsequent pollen season during which the assessment of combined symptom/medication scores, expressed as median area under the curve, showed a significant benefit for the group treated with the recombinant hypoallergenic preparation by comparison with placebo with a score of 207.8 as opposed to 389.6. A sub-group of asthmatic subjects showed an even larger reduction in combined SMS. Strong allergen specific IgG4 antibody responses were observed in all subjects that received active treatment and no serious drug related events occurred. Further studies with this recombinant Bet v 1 folding variant are in progress.

5 Recombinant Cat Allergen Fel d 1

A recombinant form of the major cat allergen Fel d 1 has been engineered to include a linker sequence between the two chains of the protein (Grönlund et al. 2003). This has in turn been fused to a TAT-derived protein translocation domain

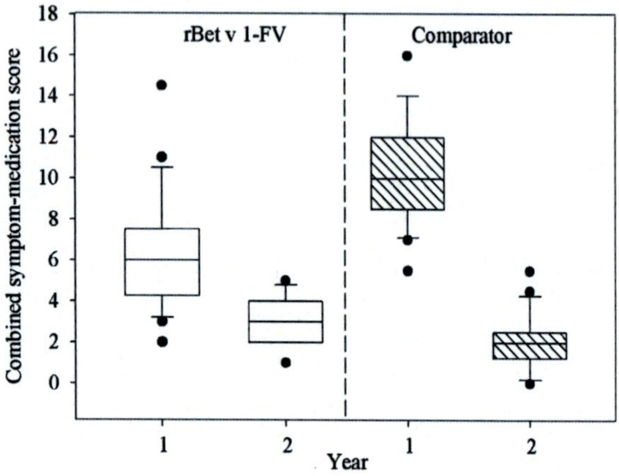

Fig. 3 Combined symptom-medication scores in birch pollen seasons following 1 or 2 years of personal subcutaneous immunotherapy with a recombinant Bet v 1 folding variant (Bet v 1-FV) or a birch pollen extract (Comparator). Boxes show median values with 25th and 75th percentiles, error bars the 10th and 90th percentiles, and points the outliers

and a truncated invariant chain for targeting the MHC class I pathway. This construct, designated MAT-Fel d 1 (Modular-Antigen-Translocation-Fel d 1), induces a shift away from a Th2 cytokine profile in cultures of human peripheral blood mononuclear cells (PBMC)(Crameri et al. 2007). This observation is supported by studies in mice which have shown that MAT-Fel d 1 stimulates higher IgG2a responses than Fel d 1 alone, leading to higher IgG2a:IgG1 ratios that are indicative of a bias toward a Th1 response (Martinez-Gomez et al. 2009). The MAT-Fel d 1 was also shown to have hypoallergenic characteristics in so far as it failed to induce anaphylaxis in sensitized mice and the stimulation of leukotriene generation by human basophils required 100-fold higher concentrations of MAT-Fel d 1 than recombinant Fel d 1 alone (Martinez-Gomez et al. 2009).

MAT-Fel d 1 has been tested in a first clinical study involving three intralymphnode injections of 1, 3 and 10 μg of the MAT-construct adsorbed to alum at four week intervals (Senti et al. 2009). Efficacy has been assessed by provocation testing, as to have various immunological parameters, but at the time of writing detailed results have not been published.

6 Ragweed Amb a 1

The major allergen of short ragweed, Amb a 1, is not as yet available as a recombinant protein for clinical studies. A purified natural Amb a 1 in combination with immunostimulatory sequences (ISS) has however been tested in the clinic (Creticos et al. 2006). These ISS bind to Toll-like receptor 9 expressed predominantly on plasmacytoid dendritic cells, and thereby mediate the down-regulation of Th2 responses. The Amb a 1 was coupled with four ISS per molecule, with the result that immunogenicity was biased in favor of a Th1 response and the allergen showed reduced IgE-binding reactivity, factors which would be considered beneficial for a more effective and safer immunotherapy (Tighe et al. 2000). A pilot study with six weekly injections prior to the pollen season showed better peak-season nasal symptom scores and improved quality of life scores by comparison with placebo (Creticos et al. 2006). There were only transient increases in allergen specific IgG, but seasonal increases in IgE were suppressed. A follow-up study gave disappointing results and the clinical development program was discontinued.

7 Where Do We Go from Here?

Recombinant DNA technology offers the prospect of a new generation of products for allergen specific immunotherapy. Products will be better defined than those derived from allergen extracts, containing highly purified active ingredients in defined concentrations that provide optimal clinical benefit. The advantages of hypoallergenic variants in respect of achieving adequate dosage and safety have already been established with chemically modified allergen extracts (allergoids), and the development of recombinant variants promises still further benefits. However it is clear that careful attention has to be paid to the selection of variants that are likely to be advantageous to a very large majority of patients selected for treatment.

The clinical development programs for products to treat some of the most common causes of allergic diseases are now gathering momentum and there are good grounds to believe that they will meet with success. The first products that are likely to be introduced on the market will provide an alternative to those derived from allergen extracts, and will be intended for the treatment of IgE sensitizations to birch and grass pollen. The prospect of recombinant products that are tailored to match the sensitization patterns to individual allergens from one source is something for the much longer term.

References

Akdis CA, Blaser K (2001) Bypassing IgE and targeting T cells for specific immunotherapy of allergy. Trends Immunol 22:175–178

Akdis CA, Blesken T, Akdis M et al (1998) Role of interleukin 10 in specific immunotherapy. J Clin Invest 102:98–106

Akdis M, Verhagen J, Taylor A et al (2004) Immune responses in healthy and allergic individuals are characterized by a fine balance between allergen-specific T regulatory 1 and T helper 2 cells. J Exp Med 199:1567–1575

Allergome (2009) A platform for allergen knowledge, http://www.allergome.org

Andersson K, Lidholm J (2003) Characteristics and immunobiology of grass pollen allergens. Int Arch Allergy Immunol 130:87–107

Breiteneder H, Hassfeld W, Pettenburger K et al (1988) Isolation and characterization of messenger RNA from male inflorescences and pollen of the white birch (*Betula verrucosa*). Int Arch Allergy Appl Immunol 87:19–24

Breiteneder H, Pettenburger K, Bito A et al (1989) The gene coding for the major birch allergen, Bet vI, is highly homologous to a pea disease resistance response gene. EMBO J 8:1935–1938
Carballido JM, Carballido-Perrig N, Terres G et al (1992) Bee venom phospholipase A2-specific T cell clones from human allergic and non-allergic individuals: cytokine patterns change in response to the antigen concentration. Eur J Immunol 22:1357–1363
Crameri R, Fluckiger S, Daigle I et al (2007) Design, engineering and in vitro evaluation of MHC class-II targeting allergy vaccines. Allergy 62:197–206
Creticos PS, Schroeder JT, Hamilton RG et al (2006) Immunotherapy with a ragweed-toll-like receptor 9 agonist vaccine for allergic rhinitis. New Engl J Med 355:1445–1455
Dahl R, Kapp A, Colombo G et al (2008) Sublingual grass allergen tablet immunotherapy provides sustained clinical benefit with progressive immunologic changes over 2 years. J Allergy Clin Immunol 121:512–518
Didier A, Malling HJ, Worm M et al (2007) Optimal dose, efficacy, and safety of once-daily sublingual immunotherapy with a 5-grass pollen tablet for seasonal allergic rhinitis. J Allergy Clin Immunol 120:1338–1345
Ferreira F, Briza P, Infuhr D et al (2006) Modified recombinant allergens for safer immunotherapy. Inflamm Allergy Drug Targets 5:5–14
Frew AJ, Powell RJ, Corrigan CJ, Durham SR (2006) Efficacy and safety of specific immunotherapy with SQ allergen extract in treatment-resistant seasonal allergic rhinoconjunctivitis. J Allergy Clin Immunol 117:319–325
Gafvelin G, Thunberg S, Kronqvist M et al (2005) Cytokine and antibody responses in birch-pollen-allergic patients treated with genetically modified derivatives of the major birch pollen allergen Bet v 1. Int Arch Allergy Immunol 138:59–66
Grönlund H, Bergman T, Sandström K et al (2003) Formation of disulfide bonds and homodimers of the major cat allergen Fel d 1 equivalent to the natural allergen by expression in *Escherichia coli*. J Biol Chem 278:40144–40151
Johansen N, Weber RW, Ipsen H et al (2009) Extensive IgE cross-reactivity towards the Pooideae grasses substantiated for a large number of grass-pollen-sensitized subjects. Int Arch Allergy Immunol 150:325–334
Juniper EF, Guyatt GH (1991) Development and testing of a new measure of health status for clinical trials in rhinoconjunctivitis. Clin Exp Allergy 21:77–83
Jutel M, Akdis M, Budak F et al (2003) IL-10 and TGF-beta cooperate in the regulatory T cell response to mucosal allergens in normal immunity and specific immunotherapy. Eur J Immunol 33:1205–1214
Jutel M, Jaeger L, Suck R et al (2005) Allergen-specific immunotherapy with recombinant grass pollen allergens. J Allergy Clin Immunol 116:608–613
Kahlert H, Weber B, Cromwell O, Fiebig H (2003) Evaluation of the allergenicity of hypoallergenic recombinant derivatives of Bet v 1 using basophil activation vy CD203c expression measurement. In: Marone G (ed) Clinical immunology and allergy in medicine. JGC Editions, Naples, pp 735–740
Kahlert H, Suck R, Weber B et al (2008) Characterization of a hypoallergenic recombinant Bet v 1 variant as a candidate for allergen-specific immunotherapy. Int Arch Allergy Immunol 145:193–206
Kettner J, Meyer H, Cromwell O et al (2007a) Specific immunotherapy with recombinant birch pollen allergen rBet v1-FV results of 2 years of treatment (Phase II trial). Allergy 62(Suppl. 83): 262 (Abstract)
Kettner J, Meyer H, Narkus A et al (2007b) Specific immunotherapy with recombinant birch pollen allergen rBet v 1-FV is clinically efficacious—results of a phase III study. Allergy 62(Suppl 83):33 (Abstract)
Klimek L, Bachert C, Doemer C et al (2005) Specific immunotherapy with recombinant birch pollen allergen rBet v1-FV is clinically efficacious. Allergy Clin Immunol Int. Suppl 1:15 (Abstract)
Larche M, Akdis CA, Valenta R (2006) Immunological mechanisms of allergen-specific immunotherapy. Nat Rev Immunol 6:761–771

Maasch HJ, Marsh DG (1987) Standardized extracts: Modified allergens–Allergoids. Clin Rev Allergy 5:89–106
Martinez-Gomez JM, Johansen P, Rose H et al (2009) Targeting the MHC class II pathway of antigen presentation enhances immunogenicity and safety of allergen immunotherapy. Allergy 64:172–178
Moverare R, Elfman L, Vesterinen E et al (2002) Development of new IgE specificities to allergenic components in birch pollen extract during specific immunotherapy studied with immunoblotting and Pharmacia CAP System. Allergy 57:423–430
Narkus A, Kniest F, Menzel A et al. (2009) Clinical trials with recombinant allergens - three perspectives: industry. Arb Paul Ehrlich Inst Bundesamt Sera Impfstoffe. Frankfurt AM 96:270–278
Niederberger V, Valenta R (2006) Molecular approaches for new vaccines against allergy. Expert Rev Vaccines 5:103–110
Niederberger V, Horak F, Vrtala S et al (2004) Vaccination with genetically engineered allergens prevents progression of allergic disease. Proc Nat Acad Sci USA 101:14677–14682
Niederberger V, Reisinger J, Valent P et al (2007) Vaccination with genetically modified birch pollen allergens: Immune and clinical effects on oral allergy syndrome. J Allergy Clin Immunol 119:1013–1019
Pauli G, Purohit A, Oster JP et al (2000) Comparison of genetically engineered hypoallergenic rBet v 1 derivatives with rBet v 1 wild-type by skin prick and intradermal testing: results obtained in a French population. Clin Exp Allergy 30:1076–1084
Pauli G, Larsen TH, Rak S et al (2008) Efficacy of recombinant birch pollen vaccine for the treatment of birch-allergic rhinoconjunctivitis. J Allergy Clin Immunol 122:951–960
Purohit A, Niederberger V, Kronqvist M et al (2008) Clinical effects of immunotherapy with genetically modified recombinant birch pollen Bet v 1 derivatives. Clin Exp Allergy 38: 1514–1525
Rappuoli R, Douce G, Dougan G, Pizza M (1995) Genetic detoxification of bacterial toxins: a new approach to vaccine development. Int Arch Allergy Immunol 108:327–333 [Review] [39 refs]
Reisinger J, Horak F, Pauli G et al (2005) Allergen-specific nasal IgG antibodies induced by vaccination with genetically modified allergens are associated with reduced nasal allergen sensitivity. J Allergy Clin Immunol 116:347–354
Ruedl C, Bachmann MF, Kopf M (2000) The antigen dose determines T helper cell subset development by regulation of CD40 ligand. Eur J Immunol 30:2056–2064
Senti G, Kuster D, Martinez-Gomez JM et al (2009) Intralymphatic allergen specific immunotherapy using modified recombinant allergen targeting the MHC class II pathway: a double-blind placebo-controlled clinical trial in cat dander allergic patients. Allergy 64(Suppl 90):74 (Abstract)
Sprung V, Pfaar O, Klimek L et al (2009) Safety and efficacy of recombinant grass pollen allergens: a dose – response study. Allergy 64(Suppl 90):147 [Abstract]
Tighe H, Takabayashi K, Schwartz D et al (2000) Conjugation of immunostimulatory DNA to the short ragweed allergen Amb a 1 enhances its immunogenicity and reduces its allergenicity. J Allergy Clin Immunol 106:124–134
Tryba M (1994) Akuttherapie anaphylaktoider Reaktionen. Ergebnis einer interdisziplinären Konsensuskonferenz. Allergo J 3:211–224
van der Heijden FL, van Neerven RJJ, van Katwijk M et al (1993) Serum-IgE-facilitated allergen presentation in atopic disease. J Immunol 150:3643–3650
van Hage-Hamsten M, Kronqvist M, Zetterström O et al (1999) Skin test evaluation of genetically engineered hypoallergenic derivatives of the major birch pollen allergen, Bet v 1: results obtained with a mix of two recombinant Bet v 1 fragments and recombinant Bet v 1 trimer in a Swedish population before the birch pollen season. J Allergy Clin Immunol 104:969–977
Vrtala S, Hirtenlehner K, Vangelista L et al (1997) Conversion of the major birch pollen allergen, Bet v 1, into two nonanaphylactic T cell epitope-containing fragments-candidates for a novel form of specific immunotherapy. J Clin Invest 99:1673–1681

Vrtala S, Akdis CA, Budak F et al (2001a) T cell epitope-containing hypoallergenic recombinant fragments of the major birch pollen allergen, Bet v 1, induce blocking antibodies. J Immunol 165:6653–6659

Vrtala S, Hirtenlehner K, Susani M et al (2001b) Genetic engineering of a hypoallergenic trimer of the major birch pollen allergen, Bet v 1. FASEB J 15:2045–2047

Weber B, Slamal H, Suck R (2003) Size exclusion chromatography as a tool for quality control of recombinant allergens and hypoallergenic variants. J Biochem Biophys Meth 56:219–232

Allergen-Specific Immunotherapy with Recombinant Allergens

G. Pauli and Hans-Jørgen Malling

Abstract Subcutaneous immunotherapy is a well-documented treatment of allergic rhinitis and asthma. The major limitation is the risk of anaphylactic side effects. The documentation of clinical efficacy is based on crude allergenic extracts sometimes containing varying amounts of individual allergens including allergens to which the patient may not be sensitized. The introduction of recombinant allergens offer a possibility to use well-defined molecules with consistent pharmaceutical quality defined in mass units. The proof-of-concept of the clinical efficacy of recombinant allergens is based on two studies published as full articles. One study applied a mixture of five *Phleum pratense* major allergens in a maximum dose of 40 μg protein. The clinical efficacy showed a significant efficacy with about 40% reduction in disease severity. The second study compared a commercial birch extract with both recombinant Bet v 1 and purified Bet v 1 in dosages of 15 μg allergen. The clinical effect was around 60% additional efficacy. Systemic side effects occurred more frequently with grass allergens. A third study used hypoallergenic fragments and a trimer of Bet v 1. The study did not show efficacy and a rather high frequency of systemic side effects. The advantages of using recombinant allergens for immunotherapy are obvious but more large-scale clinical studies are needed before the overall value in terms of efficacy and safety can be determined.

G. Pauli
Faculté de médecine, Université de Strasbourg, Strasbourg, France

H.-J. Malling (✉)
Allergy Clinic 4222, National University Hospital, Blegdamsvej 9, 2100 Copenhagen, Denmark
e-mail: all-unit@rh.dk

Current Topics in Microbiology and Immunology (2011) 352: 43–54
DOI: 10.1007/82_2011_125

Published Online: 15 March 2011

Contents

1 Introduction

Allergen-specific immunotherapy has traditionally been based on the administration of allergenic extracts containing natural allergens. These extracts are complex mixtures of allergens, and not all are well characterized and almost no standardization between different manufacturers exists. The development of recombinant allergens allow the use of well-defined allergen extracts with consistent pharmaceutical quality, in defined mass units of major allergens (van Ree et al. 2008). Non-allergenic proteins and impurities are excluded. During the last decade the potential advantages of using genetic engineering in improving both diagnosis and specific treatment has been advocated (Valenta and Niederberger 2007; Vrtala 2008). Animal experiments indicate that it is possible to convert important allergens into hypoallergenic derivatives that have the potential to be safe immunotherapeutic agents as they exhibit decreased IgE-binding capacity, contain T cell epitopes and induce IgG antibodies (Ferreira et al. 2002; Vrtala et al. 2004). However, before recombinant allergens and hypoallergenic derivatives can be considered for immunotherapy in allergic patients their immunogenic properties must be evaluated in vivo. The value of a new allergenic product in terms of efficacy and safety must be demonstrated in double-blind, placebo controlled, randomized studies (optimally in comparative studies including natural extracts) and by the use of appropriate statistical methods. This review validates clinical studies with recombinant wild-type allergens as well as recombinant hypoallergenic derivatives.

2 Strategies for Improving Efficacy of Allergen-Specific Immunotherapy

Research for candidate molecules for immunotherapy has been intense during the last decade. Two approaches are obvious. In monosensitized patients like birch pollinosis, with a dominant major allergen (Bet v 1), the use of the disease eliciting allergen only in recombinant form is applicable. In grass pollinosis with several important allergens, the use of a cocktail of recombinant allergens is another approach. Since the mid-1990s a lot of scientific work has focused on engineering allergenic molecules with reduced IgE reactivity in order to improve the safety of subcutaneous immunotherapy. As the mechanisms underlying successful immunotherapy is only partly understood, several approaches have been investigated. T cell epitope-derived peptides, from a single allergen which can induce T cell non-responsiveness as demonstrated with T cell épitopes derived from Fel d 1 (Briner et al. 1993), from Der p 1 (Hoyne et al. 1993), from Cry j 1 and Cry j 2 (Hirahara et al. 2001) have been investigated. Other approaches include hypoallergenic variants with an altered tertiary structure obtained by making mutations and deletions in allergens around B cell épitopes (IgE-binding) areas as shown for Der f 2 (Takai et al. 1997), Bet v 1 (Ferreira et al. 1998; Holm et al. 2004), Lol p 5 (Swoboda et al. 2002), Hev b 6 (Drew et al. 2004), Par j 1 (Orlandi et al. 2004), Ole e 1 (Mazaruela et al. 2006).

The limitations of natural allergenic extracts for subcutaneous immunotherapy are predominantly related to the inclusion of numerous poorly defined epitopes to which the patient may not be sensitive (but may become sensitized), a lack of or insufficiency in important allergens, and variation in allergen potencies and ratios (Valenta and Niederberger 2007). In terms of standardization regulatory authorities have problem with defining allergenic extracts as modern drugs (Geißler 2006). Molecular biotechnology made it possible to clone allergens in the early 1990s (Valenta et al. 1991, 1992). A number of concerns were however raised as to the applicability of recombinant allergens for both diagnosis and therapy. In diagnosis a major problem is related to mimicking the properties of natural allergens (an intact three-dimensional structure is critical for the IgE-binding), which may not be important for immunotherapy (Adkis and Adkis 2009). Another question is related to whether a limited spectrum of recombinant allergens is useful for immunotherapy in patients with multiple sensitivities (Vrtala 2008). Based on experiences with T-cell epitopes, the conformational structure of allergens may not be important in immunotherapy (Norman et al. 1996; Oldfield et al. 2002).

3 Clinical Trials

Despite all the promising experimental work and the potentials (Valenta and Niederberger 2007), the number of clinical trials with recombinant allergens is rather limited. Only two studies (published in full length in peer-reviewed journals) have been performed with wild-type recombinant allergens, one with a cocktail of five recombinant allergens from grasses (Jutel et al. 2005), and one with rBet v 1 (Pauli et al. 2008), and a single study performed with hypoallergenic derivatives of Bet v 1, including two groups treated with either a trimer or a mix of two fragments of Bet v 1 (Purohit et al. 2008). A study using a folding variant of

Bet v 1 published as an abstract only is not considered in this review (Klimek et al. 2005).

4 Clinical Efficacy and Side Effects of Recombinant Allergens

Clinical efficacy can be estimated by the clinical symptoms, as the primary outcome (different symptom scores can be included, i.e., the nose, the eyes, and the respiratory tract). As the total burden for the patients is a combination of symptoms and the need for rescue drugs, medications need to be taken into account to give a complete picture of the disease-reducing capacity of immunotherapy. Medication score giving a differentiated weight to the drugs used according to their relative potency (corticosteroids score higher than anti-histamines) should be included in the primary outcome. Either symptom score and medication score could be handled individually and then combined to a common score or they could be scored globally as a total symptom score (Canonica et al. 2007). Skin tests, conjunctival, and nasal provocation tests are used in some studies as secondary end-points, they are performed before therapy, after the first pollen season and/or 1 year after beginning the immunotherapy injections. Activity of an allergenic extract used for immunotherapy may be evaluated by clinical and biological markers: modification of cutaneous tests, modification of specific IgG (especially IgG1 and IgG4), specific IgE. Cytokine production was evaluated in some studies.

4.1 Recombinant Grass Allergen Immunotherapy

The first study using recombinant allergens for subcutaneous immunotherapy, was performed by Jutel et al. (2005). The study included adults (21–30 years) grass pollen allergic rhinitics (not excluding mild asthma). A total of 64 subjects were enrolled and 62 randomized to treatment, the "intention-to-treat" (ITT) population. The "per-protocol" (PP) population consisted of 29 actively treated and 28 placebo treated patients. Treatment was continued for approximately 20 months and efficacy evaluated during the second grass pollen season (defined as the 42-day period encompassing the main pollen exposure). The immunotherapy preparation used was a mixture of five Phleum pratense-derived allergens given in a maximum dose of 40 μg total protein (10 μg Phl p 1, 5 μg Phl p 2, 10 μg Phl p 5a, 10 μg Phl p 5b, 5 μg Phl p 6).

The clinical efficacy is published as both, individual score and combined score. Based on the ITT-population, the symptom score did not reach statistical significance. However, based on the PP-population, the median difference between actively treated and placebo was 37% for symptom score and 37% for medication score. The combined score showed a 39% ($P = 0.44$) reduction in disease severity for actively treated patients compared to placebo. As a secondary outcome, a rhinitis quality of life questionnaire (Juniper and Guyatt 1991) was used, and differences exceeding 0.5 score was observed for the domains "total", "activities", "non-hay fever symptoms", "practical problems", "nasal symptoms", "eye symptoms" and "emotional" in the ITT-population.

Active treatment induced a statistically significant increase in IgG1 and IgG4 *Phleum pratense* specific antibodies. Specific *Phleum pratense* IgE levels decreased significantly in actively treated with no change in the placebo group. No patients developed IgE antibodies to Phl p 5a/b despite four actively treated patients did not had an IgE-response to this allergen before immunotherapy.

Systemic side effects were observed in 7 out of 29 actively treated (24%). These include two cases of generalized urticaria (one with additional dyspnea), two cases of local urticaria, one case of rhinoconjunctivitis and one with asthma.

4.2 Recombinant Birch Allergen Immunotherapy

The second study using wild-type recombinant allergen, compared treatments performed with molecular compounds (natural and recombinant Bet v 1) with treatments performed with a commercial birch pollen extracts and placebo (Pauli et al. 2008). It showed for the first time that the efficacy of immunotherapy with a molecular allergen was at least equal to treatment with allergenic extracts containing natural allergens. A total of 165 subjects were screened and 147 randomized to treatment after a baseline season (randomized based on minimization taking symptom severity and degree of birch sensitization into consideration), the ITT-population (due to 13 discontinued before receiving any treatment) consisted of 134 adults aged 18–50 years suffering from birch pollen-induced rhinitis and possible mild asthma. Patients were randomized to four groups receiving either placebo, a commercial birch pollen extract, rBet v 1, or purified natural Bet v 1. The PP-population consisted of 33 (first year); 29 (second year) placebo treated, 28 (first year); 25 (second year) receiving birch pollen extract, 27 (first year); 25 (second year) treated with rBet v 1 and 24 (first year) and 24 (second year) nBet v 1 treated patients. Treatment was continued for 2 years and efficacy evaluated during both birch pollen seasons (defined as the period between the first and the last day with at least 40 grains/m^3/24 h). The immunotherapy schedule included after a build-up phase monthly injection of 15 μg Bet v 1 allergen or placebo.

The clinical efficacy is published as individual daily symptom score and rescue medication score. Based on the ITT-population, the mean difference between actively treated and placebo was 48% for birch pollen extract, 49% for rBet v 1 and 58% for nBet v 1 with respect to symptom score and 67% for birch pollen extract, 64% for rBet v 1 and 64% for nBet v 1 for medication score during the first season after 6 months of treatment. Figure 1a and b shows the daily rhiniconjunctivitis score and medication score during the first treatment season. Combining symptom and medication scores (equivalent weight) indicate a 59% reduction in disease severity in patients treated with birch pollen extract, 57% for rBet v 1 and

Fig. 1 **a** Mean daily rhinoconjunctivitis symptom score during the 2004 birch pollen season. The *yellow line* represents placebo-treated patients, the *red line* rBet v 1, *blue line* nBet v 1 and the *green line* birch pollen extract. **b** Mean daily rescue medication score during the 2004 birch pollen season. The *yellow line* represents placebo-treated patients, the *red line* rBet v 1, *blue line* nBet v 1 and the green line birch pollen extract

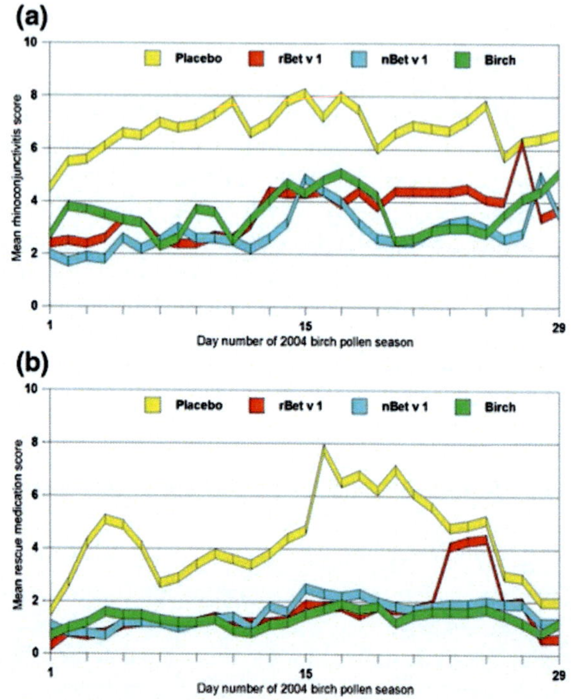

57% for nBet v 1 compared to placebo. Statistical analysis indicate no difference in symptom and rescue medication reduction between the three actively treated groups. Identical results were obtained during the second birch pollen season.

Active treatment induced a statistically significant increase in IgG1, IgG2, and IgG4 Bet v 1 specific antibodies of identical value in the three actively treated groups. Three patients in the birch pollen extract group developed de novo IgE antibodies to Bet v 2. No new sensitizations to Bet v 2 was observed in the r- and nBet v 1-treated groups. Skin sensitivity (as estimated by SPT wheal diameter) decreased to half size (identical for first and second treatment year) in actively treated patients (no change in placebo-treated patients).

Systemic side effects were observed almost equally in all actively treated (most mild reactions were almost as common in the placebo group). One patient in the nBet v 1 group developed anaphylaxis with urticaria and hypotension. Local reactions at the injection site occurred more frequently in the rBet v 1 group.

4.3 Recombinant Birch Allergen Derivatives Immunotherapy

The second study using recombinant birch pollen allergen compared treatments performed with molecular modified derivatives of recombinant Bet v 1 compared to placebo (Purohit et al. 2008). A total of 124 subjects were randomized to treatment; the ITT-population aged 23–57 years suffering from birch pollen-induced rhinitis and possible mild asthma. Patients were randomized to three groups receiving placebo, rBet v 1a trimer (created by expressing three copies of the gene in sequence) Bet v 1 fragments (two recombinant peptides that together represent the whole sequence of Bet v 1). The ITT-population consisted of 49 placebo treated, 37 treated with rBet v 1 trimer and 38 Bet v 1 fragments treated patients. The PP-population was reduced to 68% of the ITT-population and consisted of 37 placebo treated, 28 treated with rBet v 1 trimer and 19 Bet v 1 fragments treated patients (only half of the randomized patients). Treatment consisted of 4–5 months preseasonal injections and efficacy evaluated during a 8-week period encompassing the whole birch pollen seasons. The immunotherapy schedule included after a build-up phase, monthly injection of 80 μg protein.

The clinical efficacy is published as a combined symptom-medication score. Based on the PP-population, there was no difference between the trimer-group and placebo and the mean difference between the fragments-treated and placebo was 28% (NS), during the birch pollen season.

Active treatment induced a statistically significant increase in IgG1 and IgG4 Bet v 1 specific antibodies (a 100-fold increase compared with baseline) in the two actively treated groups. No significant difference in skin sensitivity and nasal challenge test between the three groups, 12 month after initiating immunotherapy was observed.

Systemic side effects related to injections were observed in both actively treated groups. Generalized urticaria was observed in 21% of fragments-treated and 16% of trimer-treated. One patient in the fragments-group developed anaphylaxis with hypotension requiring epinephrine, one generalized urticaria with severe gastro-intestinal disorders. Secondary systemic reactions occurred equally during the build-up phase or the maintenance phase; only five adverse general reactions out of 28 appeared within 30 min.

5 Discussion

Avoidance of side effects is essential if new therapeutic products are introduced. On the other hand using a safe immunogenic product that has no clinical efficacy is nonsense. According to the World Allergy Organization recommendations (Canonica et al. 2007) the magnitude of efficacy should be established as the percentage of reduction of the global clinical scores in the active versus placebo group. Additional efficacy inferior to the one established by antihistamines is not considered acceptable, and consequently the minimal clinically relevant efficacy should be at least 20% higher than placebo—and be statistically significant (Canonica et al. 2007). Based on the three published studies, applying recombinant allergens either as wild-type or hypoallergens that exhibit reduced activity by genetic engineering, the magnitude of the additional efficacy (combined symptom-medication scores) is illustrated in Fig. 2.

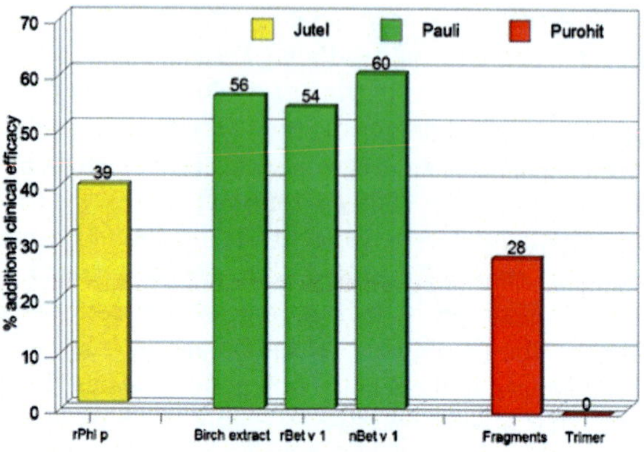

Fig. 2 The magnitude of efficacy determined as the additional clinical efficacy compared to placebo. The *yellow bar* represents data from Jutel et al. (2005) using a mixture of recombinant *Phleum pratense* allergens. *The green bars* show data from Pauli et al. (2008) comparing a crude birch pollen extract, recombinant Bet v 1 and a purified natural Bet v 1 allergen. The *red bars* present the study by Purohit et al. (2008) using fragments and a trimer of recombinant Bet v 1

5.1 Clinical Efficacy and Safety of Recombinant Allergens

In the design of the recombinant Phl p study (Jutel et al. 2005), it was planned to include 80 patients in order to ensure a sufficient power of the study. Only 62 patients were included in the ITT-population, and although the data from the PP-population (57 patients) just managed to show statistical clinical efficacy ($P = 0.44$), the magnitude of the additional efficacy was as high as 39% (for the ITT-population, the additional efficacy was also 39% but not significant). The explanation for the latter may relate to a wide variation in the individual scoring of patients. The value of the treatment is reinforced by the excellent improvement in quality of life. The study clearly documented the general view, of pure allergens being safer than crude extracts is not correct. Systemic reactions in 24% of the patients is higher than that published for natural allergens (Malling 1998). The high frequency of the systemic side effects may be related to the rather high dose of allergens injected (40 μg rPhl p) (Bousquet et al. 1998).

The rBet v 1 study (Pauli et al. 2008) not only confirm the proof-of-concept of the clinical efficacy of recombinant allergens, but also (for the birch system) that recombinant allergens are as clinically effective as purified allergen and the crude allergen extract. The magnitude already after 6 months of treatment in the order of 60% additional efficacy is very impressive (and the efficacy is consistent during the second season). The clinical results were obtained with a rather modest dose of Bet v 1 (15 μg), which may also be of importance in the low frequency of severe systemic reactions (only one patient developed anaphylaxis).

5.2 *Clinical Efficacy and Safety of Recombinant Hypoallergenic Derivatives*

The development plan behind the investigation of hypoallergenic derivatives of Bet v 1 (Purohit et al. 2008) was very ambitious at a time where the potential efficacy of rBet v 1 was not documented. However, the idea was to investigate the potential of a safer (and effective) immunotherapy by avoiding IgE-binding allergens in order to reduce the risk of inducing IgE-mediated side effects while retaining the therapeutic potential. A major problem in the study is the high number of drop-outs (in one of the centers, half of the patients were lost during the study). Power calculation is not presented and the low number of participants in the actively treated groups is a major obstruction for demonstrating clinical efficacy. The symptom score is reduced in both the fragments and the trimer group (58% for fragments and 44% for trimer) but it seems that this is caused predominantly by increasing the intake of rescue medication (almost 50% more than placebo in both the fragments group and the trimer group). Of special interest is the finding that a molecule consisting of three consecutive Bet v 1 molecules were completely without clinical efficacy based on the primary outcome—the combined symptom–medication score. The authors try to explain the deficiency of efficacy by a very low pollen count in one of the centers, but when looking at data from the other two centers, the magnitude of efficacy become even poorer (20% for the fragments). Looking at the immunogenicity based on the increase in IgG1 and IgG4, both the fragments and the trimer are able to stimulate the immune system. The clinical results from this study clearly indicate that induction of IgG-antibodies alone is not responsible for the clinical efficacy. This may be related to not differentiating between immunoreactive IgG4 (as estimated by ELISA) and functional inhibitory IgG4 antibodies (inhibition in vitro of IgE-facilitated allergen presentation) (James and Durham 2008).

Despite the anticipation that hyporeactive derivatives of Bet v 1 should be less allergenic (as documented by skin and provocation testing) (van Hage-Hamsten et al. 1999, 2002; Pauli et al. 2000) the frequency of systemic side effects is considerably higher than that in the wild-type recombinant studies. The comparisons of the rate of systemic reactions by sensitivity to Bet v 1 (evaluated by skin prick tests with different dilutions of Bet v 1 and measurement of specific IgE to Bet v 1 at inclusion in the trial) indicated that patients who experienced systemic side effects were not significantly more sensitive to Bet v 1 than those without systemic side effects. Kruskal–Wallis' test (results not published) showed no statistically significant difference in IgE variations, nor in changes in IgG1 and IgG4. No statistically significant difference in occurrence of allergen specific IgE to either trimer of fragments were observed between the group with and without side effects. This may indicate (together with the observation that most of the side effects appeared later than 1 h after injection that these side effects were not IgE-mediated.

5.3 Future Perspectives

As a proof-of-concept, the clinical efficacy of recombinant allergens has been shown. For the birch system this was to be anticipated as Bet v 1, is a very dominating allergen responsible for the majority of the birch pollen allergen activity (Niederberger and Pauli 1998). The study of the mixture of five different grass pollen allergens indicate that this may be essential for obtaining clinical efficacy in grass pollen allergics. A study using only one grass allergen would be of interest, but would likely not be effective. From a regulatory point of view (Paul-Ehrlich) licensing a single allergen would not represent major problems, but the idea of tailor-made mixtures of recombinant allergens according to the patient's sensitization profile (Valenta and Niederberger 2007; Vrtala 2008) will be a challenge to Regulators (Pfleiderer 2006). To further develop recombinant allergens for subcutaneous immunotherapy, we need to see more studies with complex allergen systems and to optimize efficacy and safety, there is an urgent need for dose-efficacy/dose-safety studies. Further investigation of hypoallergenic recombinant molecules might improve the safety of subcutaneous immunotherapy. An additional advantage of using defined molecules instead of crude allergen extract-based mixtures might be an opportunity to investigate further and more precisely the mechanisms underlying immunotherapy.

Recombinant allergens are also being applied for the sublingual mode of administrating immunotherapy. Presently a phase III study is being conducted with recombinant Bet v 1, and the results seem promising.

6 Conclusions

The two clinical trials performed with wild-type recombinant allergens have demonstrated both the clinical efficacy and the immunogenic power of genetically engineered allergens. The single study with hypoallergenic recombinant allergenic molecules show interesting perspectives, but the final form has not been achieved as no clinical efficacy has been achieved. The occurrence of side effects point out the difficulty in determining the maximum tolerated doses of molecules thought to be hypoallergenic. This cannot be predicted by previous in vitro studies or by cutaneous tests performed in sensitized patients contrary to many hopeful ideas. Even if the content of the extracts using modified hypoallergenic proteins are accurately known it remains necessary to perform clinical studies assessing clinical responses and adverse reaction rates related to different dosage regimens.

References

Adkis CA, Adkis M (2009) Mechanisms and treatment of allergic disease in the big picture of regulatory T-cells. J Allergy Clin Immunol 123:735–746

Bousquet J, Malling HJ, Locket RF (1998) World Health Organization Position Paper. Allergen immunotherapy: therapeutical vaccines for allergic diseases. Allergy 53(Suppl 54):1–15

Briner TJ, Kuo M, Keating KM, Rodgers B, Greenstein J (1993) Peripheral T-cell tolerance induced in na and primed mice by sub-cutaneous injection of peptides from the major cat allergen Fel d 1. Proc Natl Acad Sci U S A 90:7608–7616

Canonica GW, Baena-Cagnani, Bousquet J et al (2007) Recommendations for standardization of clinical trials with allergen specific immunotherapy for respiratory allergy. A statement of a World Allergy Organization (WAO) taskforce. Allergy 62:317–324

Drew AC, Eusebius NP, Kenins L et al (2004) Hypoallergenic variants of the major latex allergen Hev b 6.01 retaining human T lymphocyte reactivity. J Immunol 173:5872–5889

Ferreira F, Ebner C, Kramer B et al (1998) Modulation of IgE reactivity of allergens by site-directed mutagenesis: potential use of hypoallergenic variants for immunotherapy. FASEB J 12:231–242

Ferreira F, Wallner M, Breiteneder H, Hartl A, Tahlmer J, Ebner C (2002) Genetic engineering of allergens: future therapeutic products. Int Arch Allergy Immunol 128:171–178

Geiβler W (2006) The European guidelines regulating allergen products and the Ph. Eur. Monograph on allergens: transformation into everyday practice. In: Kurth R, Haustein D (eds) Regulatory control and standardization of allergenic extracts. GIT Verlag, Darmstadt

Hirahara K, Tatsuta T, Takatori T, Ohtsuki M, Kirinaka H, Kawaguchi J et al (2001) Preclinical evaluation of an immunotherapeutic peptide comprising 7 T-cell determinants of Cry j 1 and Cry j 2, the major Japanese cedar pollen allergens. J Allergy Clin Immunol 108:94–100

Holm J, Gajhede M, Ferreras M et al (2004) Allergy vaccine engineering: epitope modulation of recombinant Bet v 1 reduces IgE-binding but retains protein folding pattern for induction of protective blocking-antibody responses. J Immunol 173:5258–5267

Hoyne GFR, O'Hehir DC, Wraith WR, Thomas WR, Lamb JR (1993) Inhibition of T cell and antibody responses to house dust mite allergen by inhalation of the dominant T cell epitope in na and sensitized mice. J Exp Med 178:1783–1788

James LK, Durham SR (2008) Update on mechanisms of allergen injection immunotherapy. Clin Exp Allergy 38:1074–1088

Juniper EF, Guyatt GH (1991) Development and testing of a new measure of health status for clinical trials in rhinoconjunctivitis. Clin Exp Allergy 21:77–83

Jutel M, Jaeger L, Suck R, Meyer H, Fiebig H, Cromwell O (2005) Allergen specific immunotherapy with recombinant grass pollen allergens. J Allergy Clin Immunol 116:608–613

Klimek L, Bachert C, Doemer C, Meyer H, Narkus A (2005) Specific immunotherapy with recombinant birch pollen allergen rBet v 1-FV is clinically efficacious. Allergy Clin Immunol Int (Suppl N1):15

Malling HJ (1998) Immunotherapy as an effective tool in allergy treatment. Allergy 53:461–472

Mazaruela EG, Rodriguez R, Barber D, Villalba M, Batanero E (2006) Hypoallergenic mutants of Ole e 1, the major olive pollen allergen, as candidates for allergy vaccines. Clin Exp Allergy 37:251–260

Niederberger V, Pauli G Grönlund et al. (1998) Recombinant birch pollen allergens (rBet v 1 and rBet v 2) contain most of the IgE epitopes present in birch, alder, hornbeam, hazel, and oak pollen: a quantitative IgE inhibition study with sera from different populations. J Allergy Clin Immunol 102:579–591

Norman PS, Ohman JL Jr, Long AA et al (1996) Treatment of cat allergy with T-cell reactive peptides. Am J Respir Crit Care Med 154:1623–1628

Oldfield WL, Larche M, Kay AB (2002) Effect of T-cell peptides derived from Fel d 1 on allergic reactions and cytokine production in patients sensitive to cats: a randomized controlled trial. Lancet 360:47–53

Orlandi A, Grasso F, Corinti S et al (2004) The recombinant major allergen of *Parietaria judaica* and its hypoallergenic variant: in vivo evaluation in a murine model of allergic sensitization. Clin Exp Allergy 34:470–477

Pauli G, Purohit A, Oster JP et al (2000) Comparison of genetically engineered hypoallergenic rBet v1 derivatives with rBet v 1 wild-type by skin prick and intradermal testing: results obtained in a French population. Clin Exp Allergy 30:1076–1084

Pauli G, Larsen TH, Rak S et al (2008) Efficacy of recombinant birch pollen vaccine for the treatment of birch-allergic rhinoconjunctivitis. J Allergy Clin Immunol 122:951–960

Pfleiderer M (2006) Marketing authorization for recombinant products in Europe. In: Löwer J, Vieths S (eds) Regulatory control and standardization of allergenic extracts. Verlag Chmielorz, Wiesbaden

Purohit A, Niederberger V, Kronqvist M et al (2008) Clinical effects of immunotherapy with genetically modified recombinant birch pollen Bet v 1 derivatives. Clin Exp Allergy 38:1514–1525

Swoboda I, de Weerd N, Bhalla PL et al (2002) Mutants of the major ryegrass pollen allergen, Lol p 5, with reduced IgE binding capacity: candidates for grass pollen-specific immunotherapy. Eur J Biochem 32:295–302

Takai T, Yokota T, Yasue N et al (1997) Engineering of the major house dust mite allergen Der f 2 for allergen-specific immunotherapy. Nat Biotechnol 15:754–758

Valenta R, Niederberger V (2007) Recombinant allergens for immunotherapy. J Allergy Clin immunol 119:826–830

Valenta R, Duchene M, Vrtala S et al (1991) Recombinant allergens for immunoblot diagnosis of tree-pollen allergy. J Allergy Clin Immunol 88:889–894

Valenta R, Vrtala S, Ebner C et al (1992) Diagnosis of grass pollen allergy with recombinant timothy grass (*Phleum pratense*) pollen allergens. Int Arch Allergy Immunol 97:287–294

van Hage-Hamsten M, Kronqvist M, Zetterstrom O et al (1999) Skin test evaluation of genetically engineered hypoallergenic derivatives of the major birch pollen allergen Bet v 1: results obtained with a mix of two recombinant Bet v 1 fragments and recombinant Bet v 1 trimer in a Swedish population before the birch pollen season. J Allergy Clin Immunol 104:969–977

van Hage-Hamsten M, Johansson E, Roquet A et al (2002) Nasal challenges with recombinant derivatives of the major birch pollen allergen Bet v 1 induce fewer symptoms and lower mediator release than rBet v 1 wild-type in patients with allergic rhinitis. Clin Exp allergy 32:1448–1453

van Ree R, Chapman MD, Ferreira F, Vieths S, Bryan D et al (2008) The CREATE project: development of certified reference materials for allergenic products and validation of methods for their quantification. Allergy 63:310–326

Vrtala S (2008) From allergen genes to new forms of allergy diagnosis and treatment. Allergy 63:299–309

Vrtala S, Focke-Tejkl M, Swoboda I, Kraft D, Valenta R (2004) Strategies for converting allergens into hypoallergenic vaccine candidates. Methods 32:313–320

Vaccine Approaches for Food Allergy

Philip Rancitelli, Alison Hofmann and A. Wesley Burks

Abstract The prevalence of food allergy appears to be increasing. Hypersensitivity reactions to foods account for significant morbidity and mortality. The current standard of care for treatment of food allergies is limited to diligent dietary avoidance and prompt pharmacotherapy should an unexpected ingestion result in a reaction. Complex interactions between dietary antigens, the gastrointestinal flora, and the gut associated mucosal system drive host immune responses towards oral tolerance or hypersensitivity. Oral tolerance is achieved by regulatory T cell suppression of immune responses and by clonal anergy. Many novel therapies to treat food allergies are currently under investigation. Most utilize antigen-specific strategies in an attempt to induce oral tolerance. Oral immunotherapy (OIT) has been the focus of much attention. Early studies had established the safety and efficacy of OIT, but its ability to induce long-term tolerance versus a state of desensitization remains to be firmly established. Nevertheless, recent advances in our understanding of oral tolerance induction has increased optimism that disease-modifying therapies for food allergies will soon be the standard of care.

Abbreviations

OIT	Oral immunotherapy
IgE	Immunoglobulin E
APC	Antigen presenting cell
MHC	Major histocompatibility complex

P. Rancitelli
Department of Pediatrics Allergy and Immunology, Ohio State University, Columbus, OH, USA

A. Hofmann · A. Wesley Burks (✉)
Department of Pediatrics Allergy and Immunology, Duke University Medical Center, Durham, NC 27710, USA
e-mail: wesley.burks@duke.edu

Current Topics in Microbiology and Immunology (2011) 352: 55–69
DOI: 10.1007/82_2011_126

Published Online: 13 March 2011

PBMC	Peripheral blood mononuclear cell
FOXP3	Forkhead box P3
IPEX	Immune dysregulation, polyendocrinopathy, enteropathy, X-linked
FAHF-2	Food allergy herbal formula 2

Contents

1 Background

Food allergy is the result of complex immune-mediated responses to food proteins. Approximately 6% of children less than 3 years of age and 4% of adults suffer from food allergies (Sicherer and Sampson 2006). However, public perception of food allergy is much higher (Woods et al. 2002). The prevalence of food allergy appears to be on the rise. Evidence suggests that peanut allergy has risen sharply, approaching epidemic proportions (Sicherer and Sampson 2007). However, there is a paucity of well-designed prospective studies to accurately define the burden of food allergies worldwide. Future studies incorporating double-blinded placebo-controlled oral food challenges, the gold standard method for diagnosing food allergies, are needed to fill this void.

Food allergy can result from multiple deviations in immune responses to food antigens. The underlying immune mechanisms of food allergies can be classified into three general categories: immunoglobulin E (IgE)-mediated (i.e. anaphylaxis and urticaria), cell-mediated (i.e. protein enterocolitis), and a combination of IgE and cell-mediated mechanisms (i.e. atopic dermatitis and eosinophilic esophagitis). In IgE mediated food allergies, patients have a break in tolerance and make IgE to food antigens. Upon subsequent ingestions of the food, IgE binds to the food antigen and causes degranulation of mast cells which results in the symptoms of anaphylaxis. Interestingly, a small number of foods account for most food allergies (cow's milk, egg, soy, wheat, seafood, and nuts). However, any food is capable of inducing an abnormal immune response.

Although a small number of foods account for most food allergies, the distribution of these food allergies differ between children and adults. Adults are more likely to have allergies to peanut, tree nuts, and shellfish while children are more likely to have allergies to cow's milk, egg, soy, and wheat in addition to nuts and shellfish (Ando et al. 2007). Also in adults, food allergies are generally persistent and lifelong. However, in children, IgE-mediated allergy to cow's milk, egg, soy, and wheat are typically outgrown in childhood (Ando et al. 2007). It was previously thought that allergies to these foods were outgrown by the age of 5, but recent reports suggest that the time to outgrow these specific food allergies may be later at age with 79% outgrowing milk allergy by age 16 (Skripak et al. 2007; Savage et al. 2007). However, childhood allergies to peanuts, tree nuts and seafood tend to persist into adulthood (Sicherer and Sampson 2007).

2 Immune Responses to Food Antigens and Mechanisms of Oral Tolerance

The lumen of the gastrointestinal tract is the largest immunologic organ in the body (Chehade and Mayer 2005). Histologically, it is characterized by a layer of connective tissue containing lymphocytes covered by a mono-layer of epithelium which lines the lumen. A number of local and systemic immunological changes take place when antigens interact with host defense mechanisms in the gastrointestinal tract. The initial host defenses against ingested antigens are nonspecific and include digestion, mucus barriers and secretion of nonspecific antimicrobial peptides called defensins (Sicherer and Sampson 2008). As antigens that survive digestion, enter the lumen of the small intestine, they are sampled by the immune system via several mechanisms (Burks et al. 2008). Dendritic cells within the lamina propria can extend arms between epithelial cells into the lumen of the gastrointestinal tract and thereby bind enteral antigens. Particulate antigens from the lumen can be presented to dendritic cells within the lamina propria by M cells associated with Peyer's patches. T cells and macrophages in the lamina propria can sample soluble antigens via either transcellular or paracellular transport by epithelial cells. Epithelial cells that express MHC class II molecules (Scott et al. 1980; Mason et al. 1981) can also present dietary antigens to T cells.

By sampling enteral antigens in the intestine, the immune system, in the presence of other stimulatory signals, may induce an immune response to the antigen. Secondary adaptive systemic responses to ingested antigens are characterized by production of antigen specific serum and mucosal antibodies as well as generation of antigen specific T cells. Although the gastrointestinal tract is capable of making immune responses to foreign food proteins, with rare exceptions, most food proteins and commensal bacteria sampled by the immune system of the gastrointestinal tract do not stimulate immune responses. Rather, a state of immunological tolerance usually prevails.

Immunological tolerance or oral tolerance occurs when humoral or cellular immune responses to a dietary antigen are suppressed following prior oral exposure to the antigen (Chehade and Mayer 2005; Faria and Weiner 2005). The mechanisms involved in oral tolerance likely evolved over time in mammals to prevent hypersensitivity to the multitude of food and microbial antigens the immune system encounters in the gastrointestinal tract. Oral tolerance is achieved by regulatory T cell suppression of immune responses, by clonal anergy and by clonal deletion. Low dose antigen exposure leads to regulatory T cell suppression, while high dose antigen exposure leads to clonal anergy or clonal deletion (Friedman and Weiner 1994). All three mechanisms likely work simultaneously (Faria and Weiner 2005) to induce oral tolerance to food antigens. Food allergy occurs when tolerance to a food is either not achieved, or when it is disrupted.

Regulatory T cells orchestrate tolerance via important suppressive cytokines such as IL-4, IL-10 and TGF-β (Chehade and Mayer 2005); $CD8^+$ suppressor T cells (Bland and Warren 1986); and $CD4^+$ helper T cells (Chen et al. 1995; Barone et al. 1995; Garside et al. 1995). The cytokine profile associated with food allergy was nicely demonstrated by (Beyer et al. 2002). Duodenal mucosal lymphocytes of children with gastrointestinal illnesses related to milk were cultured with milk in vitro. Stimulation of these lymphocytes with milk protein resulted in the production of the T_H2 cytokines IL-5 and IL-13, while IL-10 and TGF- β expression was relatively low.

Regulatory T cells likely play an important role in the development of tolerance when a food allergy is outgrown. In a study of children with non IgE-mediated cow's milk allergy, those children who outgrew their allergy had higher levels of $CD4^+CD25^+$ T cells and reduced in vitro responses to bovine β-lactoglobulin in peripheral blood mononuclear cells (PBMCs) than children with persistent allergy. Interestingly, an increased in vitro response to β-lactoglobulin occurred in the PBMCs collected from children who outgrew the allergy following removal of $CD25^+$ cells (Karlsson et al. 2004).

Because of the likely importance of regulatory T cells in establishing oral tolerance, poor regulatory T cell activity is probably a contributing factor to the development of food allergy. The transcription factor, forkhead box P3 (FOXP3), is expressed on $CD4^+CD25^+$ regulatory T cells (Khattri et al. 2003; Fontenot et al. 2003). FOXP3 is thought to block development of both T_H1 and T_H2 immune responses (Ostroukhova et al. 2004), and mutations in the gene encoding FOXP3 result in immune dysregulation, polyendocrinopathy, enteropathy, X-linked (IPEX) syndrome (Bennett et al. 2001). Food allergy is associated with a variant of IPEX that is caused by a deletion in the noncoding region of FOXP3 that impairs mRNA splicing. This variant of IPEX I is also characterized by severe enteropathy and atopic dermatitis (Torgerson et al. 2007). Because of the involvement of mutations in FOXP3 in IPEX syndrome with food allergy, it seems possible that children with food allergies may have disruptions in T cell regulatory activity.

In addition to T regulatory cells, tolerance may also be mediated by clonal anergy or by clonal deletion. Anergy, or T cell nonresponsiveness, happens when T cell receptor ligation occurs in the absence of co-stimulation by either cytokines such as IL-2, or by lack of CD28 interaction with CD80 and CD86 on APCs (Appleman and Boussiotis 2003). Reactive T cells may also undergo apoptosis through FAS–FAS ligand interactions leading to activation induced cell death (Chen et al. 1995). Clonal deletion, or apoptosis, seem to occur in the setting of ingestion of high doses of antigens while induction of regulatory T cells seem to occur in the setting of low doses of antigen ingestion.

Given our current understanding of the mechanisms of oral tolerance, the possibility of inducing oral tolerance in allergic patients seem feasible. In fact, induction of tolerance to prevent allergy is not a novel concept. In the early 1800s, it was reported that Native Americans consumed poison ivy leaves to reduce the risk of contact reactions to urushiol (Dakin 1829). In the early 1900s, it was reported (Wells 1911) that guinea pigs did not experience anaphylaxis with injection of hen's egg protein following ingestion of it on a regular basis. By the mid-1900s (Chase 1946) reports showed that giving an antigen orally can suppress immune responses by activating T cell responses. In these studies, mice that were immunized subcutaneously responded to subcutaneous boosting with the same antigen with robust in vitro humoral and cell-mediated immune responses. However, mice fed with the antigen and boosted subcutaneously, showed blunted in vitro responses. Furthermore, when T cells were transferred from mice fed orally with the antigen to naïve mice; decreased in vitro immune responses were observed with subcutaneous immunization. The success of these animal studies suggest that induction of oral tolerance in the allergic patient may be feasible.

3 Therapeutic Approaches

The treatment options for food allergy are relatively limited in scope despite the success of immunomodulatory therapies for other allergic disorders. Treatment of hayfever with immunotherapy has been a successful therapeutic approach for years (Noon and Cantab 1911; Freeman 1930) and strong evidence supports the use of venom immunotherapy for Hymenoptera sensitivity (Hunt et al. 1978; Golden et al. 1980).

The current standard of care for managing food allergies is diligent avoidance of the suspected allergic trigger and prompt pharmacotherapy if an allergic reaction occurs. Accidental ingestions of known food triggers are unfortunately common (Yu et al. 2006). Avoidance of specific foods can be arduous for many reasons including the ubiquitous nature of common food allergens and the risk of food cross-contamination. Food avoidance can result in dietary limitations and nutritional deficits, especially for children who must avoid multiple foods. There are many social implications to avoiding foods as well. As for treatment of reactions, administration of epinephrine has associated risks, and severe reactions might not respond to pharmacotherapy.

Because of the difficulty in following elimination diets and the danger of accidental ingestion and reactions to foods, vaccination for food allergies would be an appropriate therapy for individuals unlikely to naturally develop tolerance. Evidence suggests it might be possible to identify individuals who are less likely to outgrow their food allergy. One group of investigators (Chatchatee et al. 2001) demonstrated this by looking at antibody binding sites on β-casein and κ-casein, two major cow's milk allergens, in milk allergic patients. The sera from a majority of older patients with cow's milk allergy recognized three of the nine IgE binding regions on β-casein and six of the eight IgE binding regions on κ-casein, while sera from younger patients failed to recognize these epitopes suggesting that persistent cow's milk allergy is associated with more antigen recognition. A subsequent study corroborated the use of epitope binding differences to predict persistence of cow's milk allergy (Beyer et al. 2005).

Recent interest in novel treatment approaches for food allergies has sparked a number of therapeutic-based studies (Table 1). Allergen-specific strategies manipulate the immune response to an allergenic food protein to induce a state of desensitization or immune tolerance. Examples include sublingual immunotherapy (SLIT), oral immunotherapy (OIT), immunotherapy with engineered proteins, peptide immunotherapy, plasmid DNA immunotherapy, and immunotherapy utilizing immune stimulatory sequences. The goal of these strategies is to allow consumption of a food without any deleterious effects. Allergen non-specific strategies target various immune mediators to dampen hypersensitivity responses to an allergenic food protein. Examples include Anti-IgE therapy, Chinese herbal medicine, and anti-cytokine treatments.

3.1 Allergen-Specific Strategies

3.1.1 Subcutaneous Immunotherapy

Subcutaneous allergen immunotherapy is associated with a variety of allergen-specific immune changes. Allergen-specific IgE initially rises, but later declines as allergen-specific IgG increases. Concomitantly, T_H2 driven immune responses change to a T_H1 phenotype. Subcutaneous peanut immunotherapy was studied (Nelson et al. 1997) in 12 patients of whom 6 were treated with peanut extract and 6 were treated with placebo. All of the treated patients, compared to patients who received placebo, were able to tolerate more peanut protein upon a subsequent double-blinded placebo-controlled peanut challenge. Peanut-specific IgG increased in the treatment group which is relevant, given that allergen specific IgG4 is postulated to act as a blocking antibody. IgG4 is known to increase during prolonged immunotherapy and may act to bind allergen, thereby inhibiting allergen binding to IgE which prevents allergic reactions. No immunological changes were observed in the placebo group. Despite demonstrable clinical efficacy, significant adverse effects were common and this method of immunotherapy for food allergies was therefore abandoned.

Table 1 Potential Therapeutic Strategies to Treat Food Allergies

Strategy	Mechanism	Benefits	Limitations	Status
Allergen-Specific Strategies				
Subcutaneous Immunotherapy	Present antigen at nonmucosal site	Efficacy wellestablished for venom and aeroallergen hypersensitivity	Significant side effects	Development not actively being pursued
Sublingual and Oral Immunotherapy	Present antigen at mucosal site	Safer than subcutaneous immunotherapy	Long-term tolerance induction uncertain	Multiple protocols under investigation
Immunotherapy with Engineered Food Proteins	Mutation of IgE binding sites prevent IgE activation but preserves T cell responses	Excellent safety profile	Difficult to engineer therapeutic proteins	Human studies planned
Peptide Immunotherapy	Peptides aren't large enough for IgE activation, but T cell responses are preserved	Safer than vaccination with entire allergen	Difficult to produce a validated vaccine	Murine studies only
Plasmid DNA Immunotherapy	Endogenous production of protein results in tolerance	Potential benefit with only one dose	Strainspecific variability in mice	Development not actively being pursued
Immunotherapy with Immune Stimulatory Sequences	Enhances Th1 responses	Increased efficacy and good side effect profile	Conjugation could alter allergen	Murine efficacy established
Allergen Non-Specific Strategies				
Anti-IgE Therapy	Prevents binding of IgE to high-affinity receptors	Could be efficacious for any food allergy	Variable responses in preliminary study	Studies on hold
Chinese Herbal Medicine	Unknown	Could be efficacious for any food allergy	Unknown	Human studies under way
Cytokine Therapies	Dampen hypersensitivity responses	Could be efficacious for any food allergy	Could alter natural immune responses that could be beneficial	Anti-IL-5 studies for eosinophilic esophagitis under way

3.1.2 Sublingual and Oral Immunotherapy

SLIT and OIT have undergone intense scrutiny recently. These strategies aim to first desensitize and then induce long-term tolerance in individuals with food allergies. Most studies utilize similar protocols in which patients are given very small amounts of antigen in a research setting with close observation for adverse effects. Patients then regularly consume the maximum tolerated amount of antigen on a regular basis at home. Clinical efficacy is often assessed with open or blinded food challenges, and serological studies are performed to assess immunological changes.

The efficacy of SLIT for treatment of hazelnut allergy was recently examined (Enrique et al. 2005). Twenty-three hazelnut allergic patients were randomized to either the active treatment group or placebo. Following treatment, efficacy was assessed by double-blinded placebo-controlled hazelnut challenges. The mean amount of tolerated hazelnut inducing symptoms increased from 2.29 to 11.56 g ($P = 0.02$) in the active group versus 3.49 to 4.14 g (not significant) in the placebo group. The active group, in contrast to the placebo group, was characterized by an increase in IgG_4 and IL-10 production.

Studies have (Patriarca et al. 2003) investigated OIT as an approach for treating an assortment of food allergies. Fifty-eight patients were treated with OIT, most with allergy to cow's milk (24), whole egg (13) or fish (10). Most patients (77%) were successfully desensitized, and when compared to control patients with food allergy, OIT patients were characterized by increased food-specific IgG_4 levels and decreased food-specific IgE levels. Other investigators (Meglio et al. 2004) treated 21 children with IgE-mediated cow's milk allergy with OIT. Desensitization was successful in 15 of the 21 children (71.4%). These children were able to consume 200 mL of cow's milk daily. Three of 21 (14.3%) were able to tolerate 40–80 mL of cow's milk daily. However, desensitization was not possible for 3 of the 21 children due to allergic symptoms with ingestion of small quantities of cow's milk. A more recent study (Buchanan et al. 2007) used a 24 month OIT protocol to treat 7 children with egg allergy. At the end of treatment, 4 of the 7 children passed a double-blinded placebo-controlled egg challenge of 10 g of powdered egg white. The remaining 3 children were partially desensitized. However, initial desensitization did not necessarily result in induction of tolerance. Of the 4 children who passed the initial challenge, only 2 passed a second challenge after 3 months off of egg OIT while consuming an egg-restricted diet.

Although these studies revealed encouraging preliminary results, they did not address the possibility of natural tolerance induction with increasing age. Another group of investigators (Rolinck-Werninghaus et al. 2005) reported results from an oral tolerance induction study involving 3 children with either cow's milk or egg allergy. After 37 to 52 week of therapy, patients tolerated either 250 mL of cow's milk or 4.5 g of egg protein. Per the protocol, 2 patients underwent a double-blinded placebo-controlled food challenge following a 2 month elimination diet. The third patient in this study discontinued maintenance daily dosing for only 2 days. All three patients developed moderate symptoms upon re-exposure to the causal food allergen, suggesting initial tolerance was not spontaneous.

A larger study of children with cow's milk or egg allergy utilized the same OIT protocol and an elimination diet control group (Staden et al. 2007). Upon follow-up food challenge, seven of 20 (35%) children in the control group demonstrated tolerance, compared to 16 of 25 (64%) of children showing some level of response in the active treatment group. Nine of 25 (36%) of children treated with OIT showed permanent tolerance, three of 25 (12%) were tolerant with regular ingestion, and 4 of 25 (16%) were considered partial responders. Allergen-specific IgE levels decreased significantly in both the active treatment and control groups. These results appear to validate the use of OIT as a more effective method to achieve oral tolerance than practicing avoidance.

In another study (Longo et al. 2008) 60 children with severe cow's milk allergy and high cow's milk-specific IgE were randomized to either specific oral tolerance induction (30) or a milk free diet (30). After 1 year, tolerance was assessed with either observed open feeding (tolerance induction group) or double-blinded placebo-controlled cow's milk challenges (milk free diet group). All children in the milk free diet group reacted upon re-exposure. Eleven of 30 (36%) of the children in the tolerance induction group became completely tolerant to cow's milk, 16 (54%) were partial responders tolerating 5–150 mL, and 3 (10%) could not complete the study because of persistent respiratory or abdominal symptoms. Specific IgE was significantly lower in half of the children in the treatment group at 6 and 12 months, but was essentially unchanged in the diet elimination group.

The validity of OIT studies has been strengthened by incorporating double-blinded protocols. A new report (Skripak et al. 2008) utilized a randomized, double blinded protocol to assess the effectiveness of OIT for cow's milk allergy. Nineteen children 6–17 years of age completed the study; 12 were randomized to treatment and 9 to placebo. The median baseline dose of cow's milk to induce symptoms was 40 mg for both groups. Upon double-blinded placebo-controlled challenges at the end of the protocol, the median dose to induce symptoms in the active group was 5,140 mg compared to 40 mg in the placebo group ($P = 0.003$). Milk-specific IgG levels increased significantly in the treatment group, but no significant changes in specific IgE levels were observed in either group.

Peanut allergy has been the focus of attention for immunotherapy due to prevalence acceleration, severity, and persistence. Investigators (Reese et al. 1999) recently reported results from an ongoing placebo-controlled peanut OIT study. Five patients received immunotherapy with peanut protein and five received placebo. Following the treatment phase, all children underwent an oral challenge with peanut flour. Upon challenge, the placebo patients tolerated a median cumulative dose of 460 mg ($\sim$1 peanut), but all patients in the active treatment group tolerated 5,000 mg ($\sim$13 peanuts) ($P = 0.008$). Mean peanut-specific IgE levels did not change significantly throughout the study period, but titrated skin tests were significantly improved in the treatment group compared to placebo.

These studies suggest OIT is safe and efficacious. However, important questions need to be answered prior to adopting OIT as standard therapy.

Larger studies incorporating randomized double-blinded protocols are needed to further assess dose and safety, in addition to the ability of OIT to induce long-term clinical tolerance. Nevertheless, this type of treatment strategy shows great promise, especially for those who are unlikely to become tolerant to a food spontaneously such as those with peanut allergy.

3.1.3 Immunotherapy with Engineered Food Proteins

Immunization with altered allergenic food proteins is a concept gaining interest. With this strategy, IgE-binding epitopes are engineered to attenuate IgE immune responses yet permit T cell stimulation. This approach has shown promise in a murine model of peanut allergy (Li et al. 2003). In this study, single amino acids were altered in the Ara h1, Ara h2, and Ara h3 binding epitopes of peanut proteins. These modified proteins were administered rectally with heat killed *E. coli* to C3H/HeJ peanut-sensitized mice. Following oral peanut challenge 10 weeks later, these mice were protected from anaphylaxis. The mice that received the largest dose showed significantly reduced production of IL-4, IL-13, IL-5, and IL-10. Production of IFN-γ and TGF-β was significantly increased. Efficacy and safety of these modified peanut proteins in humans remain to be elucidated.

3.1.4 Peptide Immunotherapy

Vaccination with a combination of small peptides that together extend across the entire native allergenic protein theoretically could preserve T cell activation while avoiding IgE-based immune responses. IgE recognizes conformational epitopes of larger peptides and proteins while T cell receptors recognize small linear peptides of 8 to 10 amino acids. By immunizing with small peptides, T cell activation could occur while IgE binding would be lost. One study utilizing this strategy in a murine model of peanut allergy suggested potential benefit (Li et al. 2001). However, production of a validated vaccine would be difficult due to the complexity of the stability and combination of multiple peptides in one vaccine (Sicherer and Sampson 2008).

3.1.5 Plasmid DNA Immunotherapy

Vaccination with allergen-encoding bacterial plasmid DNA is an interesting strategy. In theory, a protein endogenously produced by a host should result in tolerance. Although this type of treatment successfully prevented peanut allergy in AKR/J mice (Roy et al. 1999), strain-dependent variable responses have been observed (Li et al. 1999) in other studies. Consequently, variability of response in humans would be a valid concern.

3.1.6 Immunotherapy with Immune Stimulatory Sequences

Yet another vaccine strategy is to use immune stimulatory sequences (i.e. CpG) to enhance Th1 responses. A group of investigators (Kattan et al. 2003) orally sensitized C3H/HeJ mice with peanut and cholera toxin, followed by either treatment with intranasal CpG or no treatment. Upon subsequent peanut challenge, none of the CpG-treated mice experienced anaphylaxis. In contrast, 67% of the untreated mice showed signs of anaphylaxis. Treated mice, compared to untreated mice, had higher body temperatures, lower levels of peanut-specific IgE, higher levels of peanut-specific IgG2a, and lower levels of IL-5 in splenocyte supernatants. CpG has also been used as an adjuvant with ovalalbumin in SLIT studies in sensitized mice. Mice that received SLIT containing CpG had elevated mucosal IgA titers in the absence of elevated IgE titers, suggesting that the addition of CpG to immunotherapy may promote a Th1 response.

3.1.7 Diet-Specific Tolerance Promotion

Perhaps intervening to promote development of tolerance early in life can be an effective strategy. This idea is based on an observation that infants in Israel who regularly consume snacks with peanut protein have a lower rate of peanut allergy than Jewish infants in the United Kingdom who are not feed peanut containing snacks (Levy et al. 2003). The Learning Early About Peanut Allergy Study is investigating the possibility of early tolerance induction by enrolling 480 children between the ages of 4 and 10 months with eczema and/or egg allergy. This cohort of children has a 20% chance of developing peanut allergy based on previous studies of patients with eczema and/or other food allergies. The participants will be randomized to either avoid peanut protein until the age of 3 or to ingest about 6 g of peanut protein per week. The development of peanut allergy at 5 years will be compared (http://leapstudy.com/study_about.html, accessed 20 April 2009).

3.2 Allergen Non-Specific Strategies

3.2.1 Anti-IgE Therapy

Anti-IgE therapy for food allergy is a reasonable strategy to treat food allergies because IgE plays an essential role in food-induced anaphylaxis. One dosing study (Leung et al. 2003) used humanized monoclonal anti-IgE, TNX-901, for patients with immediate hypersensitivity to peanut using a double-blinded placebo-controlled protocol. Patients who received 450 mg of TNX-901 had significantly increased thresholds of reaction from 178 mg (~½ peanut) at baseline to 2.8 g (~9 peanuts) ($P < 0.001$) of peanut flour during oral challenge.

However, individual responses were inconsistent and not all patients would likely be protected from peanut induced anaphylaxis while on monoclonal IgE.

3.2.2 Chinese Herbal Medicine

Another treatment strategy for food allergy is the use of Chinese herbal medicine. Although the primary mechanism of action of Chinese herbal medicine is not clear, it is gaining acceptance as a legitimate treatment strategy for allergic disorders based on results of animal studies. In one particular study (Srivastava et al. 2005) the effects of food allergy herbal formula 2 (FAHF-2), a combination of specific Chinese herbs, on peanut allergic mice was investigated. Sensitized mice were treated for 7 weeks with either FAHF-2 or placebo and then challenged at weeks 1, 3, or 5 post therapy. All placebo treated mice exhibited signs of anaphylaxis and elevated plasma histamine levels following challenges. However, FAHF-2-treated mice showed no signs of anaphylaxis or significant changes in plasma histamine levels. Treated mice showed significantly lower serum peanut-specific IgE levels as long as 5 weeks post therapy. Splenocyte stimulation in vitro with peanut protein resulted in significantly lower levels of IL-4, IL-5, and IL-13 and higher levels of IFN-γ in treated mice. Although mechanistically this strategy is not well-defined, it clearly deserves further attention as a potential therapeutic approach in humans, given the promising results seen in murine studies.

3.2.3 Cytokine Therapies

Manipulation of cytokine levels might diminish hypersensitivity responses to foods. In one study of cytokine therapy, investigators (Frossard et al. 2007) transfected *Lactococcus lactis* to secrete murine IL-10. They then administered the IL-10 to young mice prior to oral sensitization with β-lactoglobulin. Administration of IL-10 resulted in significantly lessened anaphylaxis upon oral challenge, in addition to dampened serum antigen-specific IgE and IgG_1 production. Another study (Ando et al. 2007) targeted TGF-β in a murine model of food allergy. Mice that were orally fed TGF-β and ovalbumin had lower antigen-specific IgE and IgG1 antibodies, T cell reactivity, and immediate-type skin reactivity compared to mice fed only ovalbumin.

4 Conclusions

As our understanding of the mechanisms of food antigen processing, food hypersensitivity and the development of oral tolerance continue to grow, it is logical to explore new therapeutic approaches to treat and/or prevent food allergies. Recent studies using novel therapeutic approaches to treat food hypersensitivity have shown promise. Further studies are needed to better understand the efficacy and safety of these treatment modalities. Vaccination strategies will require further investigation to determine whether long-term tolerance can be induced, versus short-term desensitization. Studies should include larger numbers of patients with double-blinded placebo-controlled protocols, and immunological changes should be further elucidated. Clearly, the implementation of these novel treatments should be limited to the research setting and not in clinical practice. However, remarkable progress within the field of food allergy treatment has increased expectations that disease-modifying therapies will be the standard of care in the not so distant future.

References

Ando T, Hatsushika K, Wako M, Ohba T, Koyama K, Ohnuma Y, Katoh R, Ogawa H, Okumura K, Luo J, Wyss-Coray T, Nakao A (2007) Orally administered TGF-beta is biologically active in the intestinal mucosa and enhances oral tolerance. J Allergy Clin Immunol 120(4):916–923

Appleman LJ, Boussiotis VA (2003) T cell anergy and costimulation. Immunol Rev 192:161–180

Barone KS, Jain SL, Michael JG (1995) Effect of in vivo depletion of CD4+ and CD8+ cells on the induction and maintenance of oral tolerance. Cell Immunol 163(1):19–29

Bennett CL, Christie J, Ramsdell F, Brunkow ME, Ferguson PJ, Whitesell L, Kelly TE, Saulsbury FT, Chance PF, Ochs HD (2001) The immune dysregulation, polyendocrinopathy, enteropathy, X-linked syndrome (IPEX) is caused by mutations of FOXP3. Nat Genet 27(1):20–21

Beyer K, Castro R, Birnbaum A, Benkov K, Pittman N, Sampson HA (2002) Human milk-specific mucosal lymphocytes of the gastrointestinal tract display a TH2 cytokine profile. J Allergy Clin Immunol 109(4):707–713

Beyer K, Jarvinen KM, Bardina L, Mishoe M, Turjanmaa K, Niggemann B, Ahlstedt S, Venemalm L, Sampson HA (2005) IgE-binding peptides coupled to a commercial matrix as a diagnostic instrument for persistent cow's milk allergy. J Allergy Clin Immunol 116(3): 704–705

Bland PW, Warren LG (1986) Antigen presentation by epithelial cells of the rat small intestine. II. Selective induction of suppressor T cells. Immunology 58(1):9–14

Buchanan A, Green TD, Jones SM, Scurlock AM, Christie L, Althage KA, Steele PH, Pons L, Helm RM, Lee LA, and Burks AW (2007) Egg oral immunotherapy for egg-allergic children. J Allergy Clin Immunol 119:199–205

Burks AW, Laubach S, Jones SM (2008) Oral tolerance, food allergy, and immunotherapy: implications for future treatment. J Allergy Clin Immunol 121(6):1344–1350

Chase MW (1946) Inhibition of experimental drug allergy by prior feeding of the sensitizing agent. Proc Soc Exp Biol 61:257–259. Ref type: Generic

Chatchatee P, Jarvinen KM, Bardina L, Vila L, Beyer K, Sampson HA (2001) Identification of IgE and IgG binding epitopes on beta- and kappa-casein in cow's milk allergic patients. Clin Exp Allergy 31(8):1256–1262

Chehade M, Mayer L (2005) Oral tolerance and its relation to food hypersensitivities. J Allergy Clin Immunol 115(1):3–12

Chen Y, Inobe J, Marks R, Gonnella P, Kuchroo VK, Weiner HL (1995) Peripheral deletion of antigen-reactive T cells in oral tolerance. Nature 376(6536):177–180

Dakin R (1829) Remarks on a cutaneous affection, produced by certain poisonous vegetables. Am J Med Sci 4:98–100

Enrique E, Pineda F, Malek T, Bartra J, Basagana M, Tella R, Castello JV, Alonso R, de Mateo JA, Cerda-Trias T, Miguel-Moncin MM, Monzon S, Garcia M, Palacios R, Cistero-Bahima A (2005) Sublingual immunotherapy for hazelnut food allergy: a randomized,

double-blind, placebo-controlled study with a standardized hazelnut extract. J Allergy Clin Immunol 116(5):1073–1079
Faria AM, Weiner HL (2005) Oral tolerance. Immunol Rev 206:232–259
Fontenot JD, Gavin MA, Rudensky AY (2003) Foxp3 programs the development and function of CD4+ CD25+ regulatory T cells. Nat Immunol 4(4):330–336
Freeman J (1930) Rush inoculation, with a special reference to hay fever treatment. Lancet 1:744–747. 1–1. Ref type: Generic
Friedman A, Weiner HL (1994) Induction of anergy or active suppression following oral tolerance is determined by antigen dosage. Proc Natl Acad Sci U S A 91(14):6688–6692
Frossard CP, Steidler L, Eigenmann PA (2007) Oral administration of an IL-10-secreting *Lactococcus lactis* strain prevents food-induced IgE sensitization. J Allergy Clin Immunol 119(4):952–959
Garside P, Steel M, Liew FY, Mowat AM (1995) CD4+ but not CD8+ T cells are required for the induction of oral tolerance. Int Immunol 7(3):501–504
Golden DB, Valentine MD, Kagey-Sobotka A, Lichtenstein LM (1980) Regimens of Hymenoptera venom immunotherapy. Ann Intern Med 92(5):620–624
Hunt KJ, Valentine MD, Sobotka AK, Benton AW, Amodio FJ, Lichtenstein LM (1978) A controlled trial of immunotherapy in insect hypersensitivity. N Engl J Med 299(4):157–161
Karlsson MR, Rugtveit J, Brandtzaeg P (2004) Allergen-responsive CD4+ CD25+ regulatory T cells in children who have outgrown cow's milk allergy. J Exp Med 199(12):1679–1688
Kattan JD, Srivastava KD, Li SM, Sampson HA (2003) Intranasal treatment with CpG oligonucleotides provides protection from anaphylaxis in a murine model of peanut allergy. J Allergy Clin Immunol 111:S206 (Abstr.). Ref type: Generic
Khattri R, Cox T, Yasayko SA, Ramsdell F (2003) An essential role for Scurfin in CD4+ CD25+ T regulatory cells. Nat Immunol 4(4):337–342
Leung DY, Sampson HA, Yunginger JW, Burks AW Jr, Schneider LC, Wortel CH, Davis FM, Hyun JD, Shanahan WR Jr (2003) Effect of anti-IgE therapy in patients with peanut allergy. N Engl J Med 348(11):986–993
Levy Y, Broides A, Segal N, Danon YL (2003) Peanut and tree nut allergy in children: role of peanut snacks in Israel? Allergy 58(11):1206–1207
Li X, Huang CK, Schofield BH, Burks AW, Bannon GA, Kim KH, Huang SK, Sampson HA (1999) Strain-dependent induction of allergic sensitization caused by peanut allergen DNA immunization in mice. J Immunol 162(5):3045–3052
Li XM, Zhang TF, Huang CK, Srivastava K, Teper AA, Zhang L, Schofield BH, Sampson HA (2001) Food Allergy Herbal Formula-1 (FAHF-1) blocks peanut-induced anaphylaxis in a murine model. J Allergy Clin Immunol 108(4):639–646
Li XM, Srivastava K, Grishin A, Huang CK, Schofield B, Burks W, Sampson HA (2003) Persistent protective effect of heat-killed *Escherichia coli* producing "engineered", recombinant peanut proteins in a murine model of peanut allergy. J Allergy Clin Immunol 112(1):159–167
Longo G, Barbi E, Berti I, Meneghetti R, Pittalis A, Ronfani L, Ventura A (2008) Specific oral tolerance induction in children with very severe cow's milk-induced reactions. J Allergy Clin Immunol 121(2):343–347
Mason DW, Dallman M, Barclay AN (1981) Graft-versus-host disease induces expression of Ia antigen in rat epidermal cells and gut epithelium. Nature 293(5828):150–151
Meglio P, Bartone E, Plantamura M, Arabito E, Giampietro PG (2004) A protocol for oral desensitization in children with IgE-mediated cow's milk allergy. Allergy 59(9):980–987
Nelson HS, Lahr J, Rule R, Bock A, and Leung D (1997) Treatment of anaphylactic sensitivity to peanuts by immunotherapy with injections of aqueous peanut extract. J Allergy Clin Immunol 99 (6 Pt 1):744–751
Noon L, Cantab B (1911) Prophylactic inoculation against hay fever. Lancet 177:1572–1573
Ostroukhova M, Seguin-Devaux C, Oriss TB, Dixon-McCarthy B, Yang L, Ameredes BT, Corcoran TE, Ray A (2004) Tolerance induced by inhaled antigen involves CD4(+) T cells expressing membrane-bound TGF-beta and FOXP3. J Clin Invest 114(1):28–38

Patriarca G, Nucera E, Roncallo C, Pollastrini E, Bartolozzi F, De Pasquale T, Buonomo A, Gasbarrini G, Di Campli C, Schiavino D (2003) Oral desensitizing treatment in food allergy: clinical and immunological results. Aliment Pharmacol Ther 17(3):459–465

Reese G, Ayuso R, Lehrer SB (1999) Tropomyosin: an invertebrate pan-allergen. Int Arch Allergy Immunol 119(4):247–258

Rolinck-Werninghaus C, Staden U, Mehl A, Hamelmann E, Beyer K, Niggemann B (2005) Specific oral tolerance induction with food in children: transient or persistent effect on food allergy? Allergy 60(10):1320–1322

Roy K, Mao HQ, Huang SK, Leong KW (1999) Oral gene delivery with chitosan–DNA nanoparticles generates immunologic protection in a murine model of peanut allergy. Nat Med 5(4):387–391

Savage JH, Matsui EC, Skripak JM, Wood RA (2007) The natural history of egg allergy. J Allergy Clin Immunol 120(6):1413–1417

Scott H, Solheim BG, Brandtzaeg P, Thorsby E (1980) HLA-DR-like antigens in the epithelium of the human small intestine. Scand J Immunol 12(1):77–82

Sicherer SH, Sampson HA (2006) 9. Food allergy. J Allergy Clin Immunol 117 (2 Suppl Mini-Primer):S470–S475

Sicherer SH, Sampson HA (2007) Peanut allergy: emerging concepts and approaches for an apparent epidemic. J Allergy Clin Immunol 120(3):491–503

Sicherer SH Sampson HA (2008) Food Allergy: Recent Advances in Pathophysiology and Treatment. Annu Rev Med 60:261–277

Skripak JM, Matsui EC, Mudd K, Wood RA (2007) The natural history of IgE-mediated cow's milk allergy. J Allergy Clin Immunol 120(5):1172–1177

Skripak JM, Nash SD, Rowley H, Brereton NH, Oh S, Hamilton RG, Matsui EC, Burks AW, Wood RA (2008) A randomized, double-blind, placebo-controlled study of milk oral immunotherapy for cow's milk allergy. J Allergy Clin Immunol 122(6):1154–1160

Srivastava KD, Kattan JD, Zou ZM, Li JH, Zhang L, Wallenstein S, Goldfarb J, Sampson HA, Li XM (2005) The Chinese herbal medicine formula FAHF-2 completely blocks anaphylactic reactions in a murine model of peanut allergy. J Allergy Clin Immunol 115(1):171–178

Staden U, Rolinck-Werninghaus C, Brewe F, Wahn U, Niggemann B, Beyer K (2007) Specific oral tolerance induction in food allergy in children: efficacy and clinical patterns of reaction. Allergy 62(11):1261–1269

Torgerson TR, Linane A, Moes N, Anover S, Mateo V, Rieux-Laucat F, Hermine O, Vijay S, Gambineri E, Cerf-Bensussan N, Fischer A, Ochs HD, Goulet O, Ruemmele FM (2007) Severe food allergy as a variant of IPEX syndrome caused by a deletion in a noncoding region of the FOXP3 gene. Gastroenterology 132(5):1705–1717

Wells H-G (1911) Studies on the chemistry of anaphylaxis III. Experiments with isolated proteins, especially those of the hens egg. J Infect Dis 8:147–171

Woods RK, Stoney RM, Raven J, Walters EH, Abramson M, Thien FC (2002) Reported adverse food reactions overestimate true food allergy in the community. Eur J Clin Nutr 56(1):31–36

Yu JW, Kagan R, Verreault N, Nicolas N, Joseph L, St Pierre Y, Clarke A (2006) Accidental ingestions in children with peanut allergy. J Allergy Clin Immunol 118(2):466–472

Intralymphatic Immunotherapy: From the Rationale to Human Applications

Gabriela Senti, Pål Johansen and Thomas M. Kündig

Abstract Allergen specific immunotherapy (SIT) is the only treatment of IgE mediated allergies that is causative and has a long-term effect. Classically, SIT requires numerous subcutaneous injections of the allergen during 3–5 years. Over the last decade sublingual allergen applications have established as an alternative, but treatment duration could not be shortened. This review focuses on direct administration of vaccines in general and of allergens in particular into lymph nodes with the aim to enhance immunotherapy. Several studies have found that direct injection of antigens into lymph nodes enhanced immune responses. Recently we have focused on intralymphatic allergen administration in order to enhance SIT. Data in mouse models and in clinical trials showed that intralymphatic allergen administration strongly enhanced SIT, so that the number of allergen injections could be reduced to three, and the allergen dose could be reduced 10–100 fold. Intralymphatic injections proved easy, practically painless and safe. In mice and men, intralymphatic immunotherapy injecting allergens into a subcutaneous lymph node markedly enhances the protective immune response, so that both the dose and number of allergen injections can be reduced, making SIT safer and faster, which enhances patient convenience and compliance.

G. Senti (✉)
Clinical Trials Center, Center for Clinical Research,
University and University Hospital of Zurich,
Rämistrasse 100, 8091 Zurich, Switzerland
e-mail: gabriela.senti@usz.ch

P. Johansen · T. M. Kündig
Department of Dermatology,
University Hospital of Zurich,
8091 Zurich, Switzerland

Current Topics in Microbiology and Immunology (2011) 352: 71–84
DOI: 10.1007/82_2011_133

Published Online: 3 July 2011

Contents

1 Introduction

1.1 The Function of Lymph Nodes

T and B cell receptors are randomly rearranged early in lymphocyte development generating T and B cells carrying a diverse repertoire of receptors. This allows for specific recognition of nearly all possible antigens, but the problem is that only 1 in 10^7 T and B cells is specific for an antigen, so that antigens must be presented to millions of T and B cells to elicit a response. Therefore antigens are drained into secondary lymphatic organs, where they can be presented to high numbers of T and B cells. Only antigens that drain into lymph nodes or are transported there elicit immune responses, whereas antigens staying outside of secondary lymphoid organs have little chance to meet with specific T or B cells and are poorly immunogenic. More than a decade ago, we called this the "geographic concept of immunogenicity" (Kundig et al. 1995; Zinkernagel et al. 1997; Zinkernagel 2000) (Fig. 1). While the current understanding of immune regulation by dendritic cells and T cells makes this concept look simplistic, it remains nevertheless valid. It must never be forgotten that the key trigger and regulator of immune response is the antigen.

The importance of antigen drainage or transport from the periphery into lymph nodes via afferent lymph vessels has been unequivocally demonstrated by elegant early skin flap experiments performed by Frey and Wenk (1957), and experiments

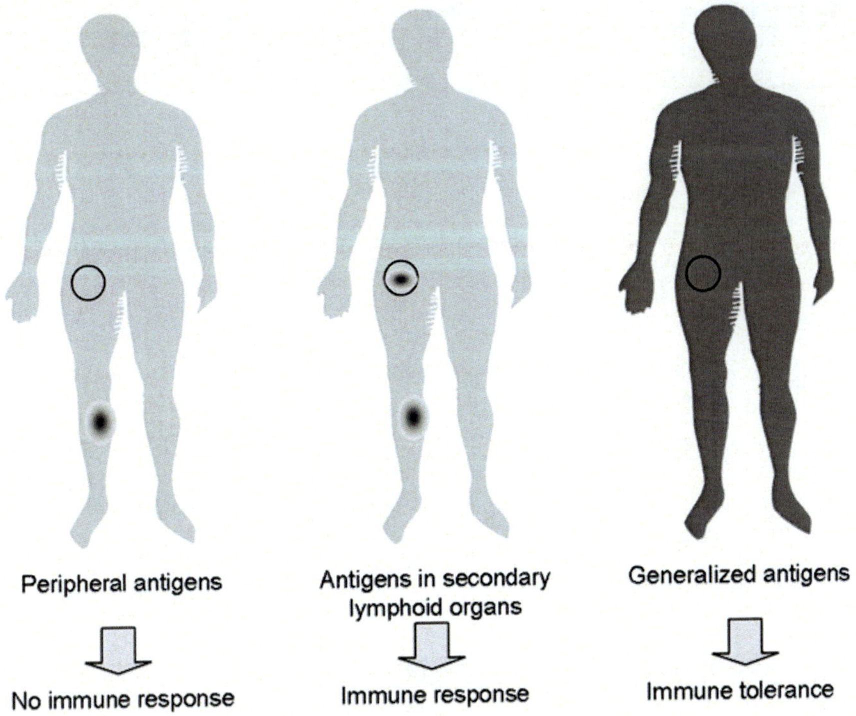

Fig. 1 Geographical concept of immunogenicity: *Left* Antigens which remain localized only in peripheral solid organs are poorly immunogenic, as pathogens with no tendency to spread typically pose no threat to the organism. *Middle* Antigens draining and replicating in lymph nodes induce a strong immune response, as such pathogens threaten to further infect the organism. *Right* Antigens distributed all over the organism are poorly immunogenic, because any immune response attempting to clear such pathogens would cause severe immunopathology

in alymphoplastic (aly/aly) and spleenless (Hox11$^{-/-}$) mutant mice confirm the importance of secondary lymphoid organs, or neo-lymphoid aggregates (Greter et al. 2009) in generating immune responses (Karrer et al. 1997).

1.2 Targeting Antigen to Lymph Nodes

Lymph vessels drain substances from the interstitial fluid into regional lymph nodes with highly variable efficiency. As lymph vessels have evolved to drain pathogens into lymph nodes, small particles sized 20–200 nm, i.e. the size of viruses, drain from peripheral injection sites into lymph nodes quite efficiently and in a free form, but even in this case usually only a few percent of the injected particles drain into the lymph nodes (Manolova et al. 2008). Larger particles sized 500–2,000 nm are mostly transported into lymph nodes by dendritic cells (DCs) (Manolova et al. 2008). Drainage from periphery to lymph nodes of non-particulate antigens,

Table 1 Intralymphatic vaccination strongly enhances unstable vaccines

Type of vaccine	Dose required s.c./intralyphatic	Stability in vivo and drainage into lymph node
Naked RNA[a]	$>10^6$	-
Oligopeptide (Johansen et al. 2005)	10^6	+
Naked DNA (Maloy et al. 2001)	10^3–10^4	++
Protein (Martinez-Gomez et al. 2009)	10^3–10^4	+++
Live virus[b]	1	++++

[a] TMK unpublished and (Kreiter et al. 2010), [b] TMK unpublished

however, can be much less efficient and only very small fractions—between 10^{-3} and 10^{-6}—of the injected doses reach lymph nodes, as discussed below and summarized in Table 1. As many of today's vaccines and immunotherapeutic agents are non-particulate, their direct administration into a lymph node may therefore markedly enhance antigen presentation in the lymph node and the immune response.

1.3 Intralymphatic Immunotherapy (ILIT) with Dendritic Cells

The vast majority of DCs injected subcutaneously or intradermally remains at the injection site (Barratt-Boyes et al. 2000; Morse et al. 1999; De Vries et al. 2003; Lesimple et al. 2003; Quillien et al. 2005; Thomas et al. 1999; Barratt-Boyes et al. 1997), so that intralymphatic and intranodal delivery of DC-based vaccines have been attempted (Lesimple et al. 2006; Mackensen et al. 1999; Grover et al. 2006). Antigen-pulsed DCs injected into the lymph node localize to the paracortex (De Vries et al. 2003; Brown et al. 2003; de Vries et al. 2005), and clinical trials have suggested that intralymphatic administration of DC vaccines enhanced immune responses (Lesimple et al. 2003). In other clinical trials, however, no advantage of intranodal delivery over intradermal delivery of DCs was found (Brown et al. 2003; Fong et al. 2001).

1.4 ILIT with Tumor Cells

As DCs and T cells are present at very high densities in lymph nodes, costimulatory signals for T and B cell induction may be provided as a bystander effect. We found that also non-professional APC, such as a fibrosarcoma cell line efficiently induced antigen specific $CD8^+$ T cell responses in lymph nodes via direct antigen presentation on the MHC class I molecule on the fibrosarcoma (Kundig et al. 1995; Ochsenbein et al. 2001). Intralymphatic immunization using tumor cells has been tried in both human cancer patients and dogs with indication of success (Juillard and Boyer 1977; Juillard et al. 1976, 1977, 1978, 1979).

1.5 ILIT with MHC Class I Binding Peptides

We found that direct administration of MHC class I binding peptides into lymph nodes (Johansen et al. 2005) or spleen dramatically enhanced $CD8^+$ T cell responses in mice, and have shown that ILIT using DNA priming followed by a peptide boost produced the strongest $CD8^+$ T cell responses that can be observed in mice with frequencies of peptide specific $CD8^+$ T cells reaching up to 80% (Smith et al. 2009).

1.6 ILIT with Naked DNA

ILIT also markedly enhanced naked DNA vaccines in mice (Smith et al. 2009; Maloy et al. 2001; Heinzerling et al. 2006). While experiments in dairy cows did not reproduce our observations, however, clinical trials on ILIT using a Melan-A/MART-1 DNA plasmid vaccine in stage IV melanoma patients generated significant immune responses correlating with tumor responses (Weber et al. 2008; Tagawa et al. 2003).

1.7 ILIT with RNA-Based Vaccines

A recent study demonstrated that administration into the lymph node strongly enhanced immunogenicity of mRNA vaccines (Kreiter et al. 2010). This pre-clinical work demonstrated that intra lymph node administration of a mRNA vaccine generated around ten-fold higher frequencies of specific T cells when compared to subcutaneous or intradermal injection, and also when compared to injection near to the lymph node. The mRNA was selectively taken up by lymph node resident dendritic cells, in particular $CD11c^+$, $CD11b^+$, and $CD11c^+$ $CD8^+$ dendritic cell subpopulations, known to be efficient stimulators of T cells.

1.8 Intralymphatic Vaccination with Vaccinia Virus

Intranodal immunization with a vaccinia virus encoding multiple antigenic epitopes and costimulatory molecules in patients with metastatic stage III and IV melanoma proved safe and immunogenic in the majority of patients, but did not prove obviously more immunogenic than intradermal administration, although this conclusion was drawn from historical data and not from a direct comparison (Adamina et al. 2010).

1.9 ILIT with ISCOMS

The intranasal route was compared to targeted lymph node immunization using HIV formulated in PR8-Flu ISCOM adjuvant in rhesus macaques. Targeting the vaccine to the lymph node was found to generate significantly stronger T and B cell responses (Koopman et al. 2007).

1.10 ILIT with Protein-Based Vaccines

ILIT was performed with proteins very early, when researchers wanted to produce antibodies against proteins of which they had been able to purify only very small amounts, and were therefore looking for the most efficient route of immunization (Sigel et al. 1983). Nanogram quantities of protein have been shown to elicit immune responses when injected into lymph nodes (Nilsson et al. 1987).

Targeted lymph node immunization is also extensively documented to be the most efficient means to immunize macaques against SIV. Vaccination using envelope gp120 and core p27 was performed by targeted lymph node immunization, via the intradermal, nasal, or intramuscular route. Only targeted lymph node immunization induced protection against the SIV challenge, whereas none of the other routes induced a protective immune response (Lehner et al. 1996). Similar results were obtained in macaques vaccinated with p27 alone (Kawabata et al. 1998), with HSP70 linked either to SIVgp120 or p27 (Lehner et al. 2000), with HSP70 conjugated to HIV gp120, SIV p27, and CCR5 peptides (Bogers et al. 2004a, b), a particulate SIVp27 protein vaccine (Klavinskis et al. 1996), or SIVp27 virus like particles (Lehner et al. 1994).

Targeted lymph node immunization also proved to be the most efficient route to immunize cats against feline immunodeficiency using virus when using a protein-based vaccine (Finerty et al. 2001), and the superior efficacy of lymph node targeting was also confirmed for protein vaccines in cows (Guidry et al. 1994).

1.11 ILIT with BCG

Julliard et al. report a comparison of intralymphatic versus intradermal vaccination with BCG, where it was found that the tuberculin test became positive more rapidly (11–23 days) after intralymphatic than after intradermal vaccination (45 days) (Juillard and Boyer 1977).

1.12 ILIT with Adjuvants

ILIT may also be used to enhance adjuvants. We found that intralymphatic administration of CpG required 100 times lower doses than subcutaneous administration, thus avoiding unwanted systemic adverse effects of the adjuvant (von Beust et al. 2005). This is in line with reports of better safety profiles and enhanced efficacy of CpG when targeted to lymph nodes using particles (Storni et al. 2004; Bourquin et al. 2008).

1.13 Inefficient Vaccines Profit the Most from Intralymphatic Administration

For various types of vaccines we have meanwhile compared the doses required when injected directly into subcutaneous lymph nodes to the doses required when subcutaneously injected (Table 1). Those vaccines that are the least stable appear to profit the most from direct intralymphatic administration. Using ILIT we could induce specific $CD8^+$ T cell responses even by injection of naked mRNA encoding for lymphocytic choriomeningitis virus (LCMV) glycoprotein, which could not be achieved even with the highest doses of mRNA by subcutaneous vaccination (TMK unpublished), obviously because RNA in tissues is rapidly digested by RNase. At the other end of the spectrum, we tried to enhance T cell responses by injection of live LCMV into a subcutaneous lymph node, but found no advantage over i.v. infection (TMK unpublished). Obviously, the virus particles efficiently drained into the lymph nodes and replicated there.

Overall, vaccines that work only poorly by subcutaneous or intramuscular administration profit the most from intralymphatic delivery, while vaccines that already induce strong immune responses after s.c. or i.m. administration may not be further enhanced (Fig. 2).

1.14 ILIT with Allergens

IgE-mediated allergies, such as allergic rhino-conjunctivitis and asthma, have become highly prevalent, and today affect up to 35% of the population in the western countries (Arbes et al. 2005; Verlato et al. 2003; ISAAC steering committee 1998; Wuthrich et al. 1996). The gold standard treatment is subcutaneous allergen-specific immunotherapy (SCIT), the administration of gradually increasing quantities of an allergen vaccine to an allergic subject, which is an effective treatment for allergic rhinitis, conjunctivitis, asthma, and allergic reactions from stinging insects (Bousquet et al. 1998; Lockey 2001; Varney et al. 1991). SCIT confers long-term benefits even after discontinuation (Durham et al. 1999; Golden et al. 1996), interrupts expansion of allergic sensitization (Pajno

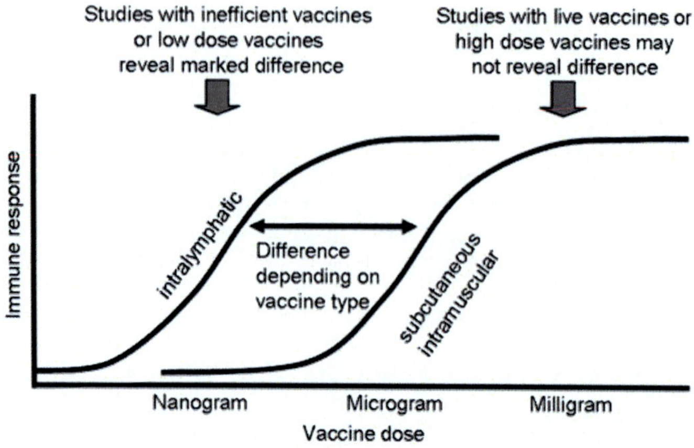

Fig. 2 Inefficient vaccines profit the most from intralymphatic delivery: High-dose vaccines which after subcutaneous or intramuscular administration already work efficiently may profit from intralymphatic administration, as they are already "maxed out". Also, live vaccines are drained into lymph nodes efficiently and may not be further enhanced by intralymphatic administration. In contrast, inefficient vaccines, e.g. subcomponent vaccines which are not of particulate nature and do not readily drain into lymph nodes, or low-dose vaccines, profit the most from intralymphatic delivery

et al. 2001) and progression from allergic rhinitis to asthma (Moller et al. 2002). From a medical perspective, SCIT is therefore superior to symptomatic treatment. However, SIT involves 30–80 allergen injections and therefore doctor visits over 3–5 years and is associated with frequent allergic side effects and with a risk of anaphylaxis and even death (Lockey et al. 1987, 1990; Stewart and Lockey 1992).

SIT acts by modulating the allergen-specific immune response, shifting the balance of T-lymphocyte subsets from a Th2 towards a Th1 phenotype with preferential IFN-γ and decreased IL-4 and IL-5 production (Till et al. 2004; Norman 2004). Also, production of allergen-specific IL-10 by $CD4^+$ $CD25^+$ T-regulatory cells is observed (Till et al. 2004; Vissers et al. 2004), and serum levels and affinity of allergen-specific IgG antibodies, especially IgG4, increase (Pierson-Mullany et al. 2000). Which one of these immunological mechanisms is ultimately responsible for ameliorating the allergy symptoms is a matter of debate.

In light of the above we investigated whether SCIT could be enhanced by intralymphatic administration. In mice, we compared the immunization efficiency of different administration routes for SIT using phospholipase-A2 (PLA2), the major allergen of bee venom. In fact, changing from the subcutaneous route to direct intralymphatic injection significantly enhanced the efficiency of immunization, inducing allergen-specific IgG2a antibody responses which were 10–20 times higher with only 0.1% of the allergen dose (Martinez-Gomez et al. 2009a).

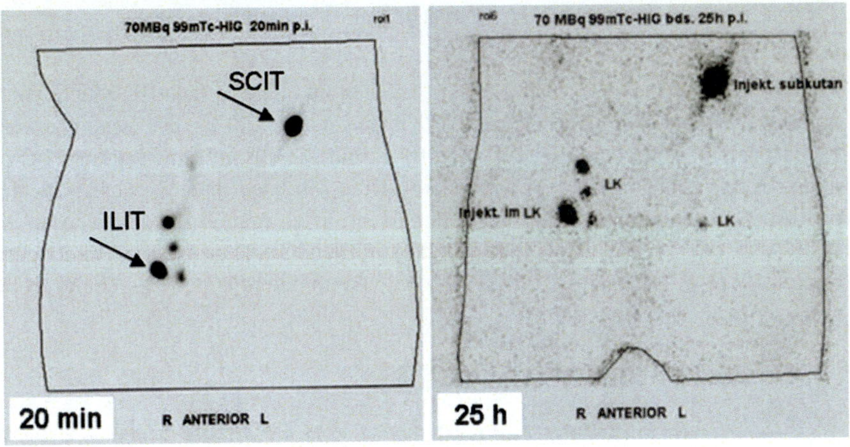

Fig. 3 Biodistribution after intralymphatic administration: Biodistribution of ^{99m}Tc-labelled human IgG after intralymphatic (*left abdominal side*) and subcutaneous (*right abdominal side*) injections. Radio tracing was made by gamma-imaging 20 min (*left panel*) and 25 h (*right panel*) after injection. Arrows indicate the site of injection (SCIT subcutaneous, ILIT intralymphatic)

Since allergic side effects are proportional to the allergen dose, intralymphatic SIT should not only show enhanced efficiency, but also reduce side effects.

In mice, intralymphatic injection of allergens enhanced IL-1, IFNγ, IL-4, and IL-10 secretion when compared to subcutaneous injection, thus Th1, Th2, and Treg responses, suggesting that ILIT did not polarize the response to the allergen, but generated overall stronger responses (Martinez-Gomez et al. 2009a).

1.15 Biodistribution After Intralymphatic Versus Subcutaneous Injection in Humans

Biodistribution studies in mice found 100-fold higher allergen doses in an injected lymph node than after subcutaneous injection into the draining region (Martinez-Gomez et al. 2009a). Similar results were obtained in humans when comparing intralymphatic to subcutaneous injection using radiotracing. On the right abdominal side a ^{99m}Tc labeled protein was injected directly into a superficial inguinal lymph node under. On the left side the same dose was injected subcutaneously, but 10 cm above the inguinal lymph nodes. Only a small fraction of the subcutaneously administered protein reached the lymph nodes after 4 hours and this fraction did not increase after 24 hours (Fig. 3). After intralymphatic injection, however, the protein drained into the deep subcutaneous lymph nodes and further into one pelvic lymph node already within 20 minutes. Thus, intralymphatic injection efficiently pulsed five lymph nodes with the full amount of the protein.

1.16 Clinical Trials on ILIT with Bee Venom

In a first clinical trial eight patients with bee venom allergy grade III, which would normally receive SCIT with approx. 70 injections of 100 μg bee venom extract each, received three injections of only 10 μg but directly into the inguinal lymph node. In this proof-of-concept trial 7 out of the 8 treated patients were protected against a subsequent bee sting challenge (Senti et al. manuscript in preparation). ILIT with bee venom also proved highly immunogenic in a larger multicenter clinical trial in 66 grade III and IV bee venom allergic patients (Senti et al. manuscript in preparation).

1.17 Clinical Trials on ILIT to Treat Pollen-Induced Hay Fever

In a monocentric open-label trial, 165 patients with grass pollen-induced rhinoconjunctivitis were randomized to receive either 54 s.c. injections with pollen extract over 3 years (cumulative allergen dose 4,031,540 standardized quality units (SQ-U)) or three intralymphatic injections over 2 months (cumulative allergen dose 3,000 SQ-U). Patients were evaluated after 4 months, 1 year, and 3 years. Three low-dose intralymphatic allergen administrations increased tolerance to nasal provocation with pollen already within 4 months. Tolerance was long lasting and equivalent to that achieved after standard s.c. immunotherapy. ILIT ameliorated hay fever symptoms, reduced skin prick test reactivity, decreased specific serum IgE, caused fewer adverse events than s.c. immunotherapy, enhanced compliance, and was less painful than venous puncture. In conclusion, intralymphatic allergen administration enhanced safety and efficacy of immunotherapy and reduced treatment time from 3 years to 8 weeks.

1.18 Future Direction

As ILIT brings the antigen into close proximity to DCs, intracellular translocation sequences and sequences further targeting the allergen molecule to the MHC class II pathway may further enhance allergen-specific immunotherapy. By fusing allergens to a tat-translocation peptide derived from HIV and to a part of the invariant chain we were able to target the allergen to MHC class II molecules located in the endoplasmatic reticulum. As this circumvents the inefficient pinocytosis process and enzymatic degradation in phagolysosomes, immunogenicity could be significantly further enhanced (Martinez-Gomez et al. 2009a, b; Rhyner et al. 2007; Crameri et al. 2007). A double blinded placebo controlled trial on ILIT using this new generation of therapeutic allergen molecules has proved the concept (Senti et al. manuscript in preparation).

1.19 Is ILIT Difficult or Painful?

In our hands ultrasound guided injection into a subcutaneous lymph node in the groin area is performed within minutes, and proved practically painless. The pain of intralymphatic injection arises solely from penetrating the skin, whereas lymph nodes are poorly innervated. The pain of an intralymphatic injection is comparable to the subcutaneous injections during conventional SIT. In fact, patients rated intralymphatic injection as less painful than venous puncture (Senti et al. 2008).

In conclusion, intralymphatic SIT allows to markedly reduce both the number and the dose of the allergen injections, thus making the treatment shorter and safer. The procedure is practically painless and enhances patient compliance (Senti et al. 2008) as only three injections instead of numerous injections over the years are necessary.

References

Adamina M, Rosenthal R, Weber WP, Frey DM, Viehl CT, Bolli M et al (2010) Intranodal immunization with a vaccinia virus encoding multiple antigenic epitopes and costimulatory molecules in metastatic melanoma. Mol Ther 18:651–659

Arbes SJ Jr, Gergen PJ, Elliott L, Zeldin DC (2005) Prevalences of positive skin test responses to 10 common allergens in the US population: results from the third national health and nutrition examination survey. J Allergy Clin Immunol 116:377–383

Barratt-Boyes SM, Watkins SC, Finn OJ (1997) Migration of cultured chimpanzee dendritic cells following intravenous and subcutaneous injection. Adv Exp Med Biol 417:71–75

Barratt-Boyes SM, Zimmer MI, Harshyne LA, Meyer EM, Watkins SC, Capuano S III et al (2000) Maturation and trafficking of monocyte-derived dendritic cells in monkeys: implications for dendritic cell-based vaccines. J Immunol 164:2487–2495

Bogers WM, Bergmeier LA, Ma J, Oostermeijer H, Wang Y, Kelly CG et al (2004a) A novel HIV-CCR5 receptor vaccine strategy in the control of mucosal SIV/HIV infection. Aids 18:25–36

Bogers WM, Bergmeier LA, Oostermeijer H, ten Haaft P, Wang Y, Kelly CG et al (2004b) CCR5 targeted SIV vaccination strategy preventing or inhibiting SIV infection. Vaccine 22:2974–2984

Bourquin C, Anz D, Zwiorek K, Lanz AL, Fuchs S, Weigel S et al (2008) Targeting CpG oligonucleotides to the lymph node by nanoparticles elicits efficient antitumoral immunity. J Immunol 181:2990–2998

Bousquet J, Lockey R, Malling HJ (1998) Allergen immunotherapy: therapeutic vaccines for allergic diseases. A WHO position paper. J Allergy Clin Immunol 102:558–562

Brown K, Gao W, Alber S, Trichel A, Murphey-Corb M, Watkins SC et al (2003) Adenovirus-transduced dendritic cells injected into skin or lymph node prime potent simian immunodeficiency virus-specific T cell immunity in monkeys. J Immunol 171:6875–6882

Crameri R, Fluckiger S, Daigle I, Kundig T, Rhyner C (2007) Design, engineering and in vitro evaluation of MHC class-II targeting allergy vaccines. Allergy 62:197–206

De Vries IJ, Krooshoop DJ, Scharenborg NM, Lesterhuis WJ, Diepstra JH, Van Muijen GN et al (2003) Effective migration of antigen-pulsed dendritic cells to lymph nodes in melanoma patients is determined by their maturation state. Cancer Res 63:12–17

de Vries IJ, Lesterhuis WJ, Barentsz JO, Verdijk P, van Krieken JH, Boerman OC et al (2005) Magnetic resonance tracking of dendritic cells in melanoma patients for monitoring of cellular therapy. Nat Biotechnol 23:1407–1413

Durham SR, Walker SM, Varga EM, Jacobson MR, O'Brien F, Noble W et al (1999) Long-term clinical efficacy of grass-pollen immunotherapy. N Engl J Med 341:468–475
Finerty S, Stokes CR, Gruffydd-Jones TJ, Hillman TJ, Barr FJ, Harbour DA (2001) Targeted lymph node immunization can protect cats from a mucosal challenge with feline immunodeficiency virus. Vaccine 20:49–58
Fong L, Brockstedt D, Benike C, Wu L, Engleman EG (2001) Dendritic cells injected via different routes induce immunity in cancer patients. J Immunol 166:4254–4259
Frey JR, Wenk P (1957) Experimental studies on the pathogenesis of contact eczema in the guinea-pig. Int Arch Allergy Appl Immunol 11:81–100
Golden DB, Kwiterovich KA, Kagey-Sobotka A, Valentine MD, Lichtenstein LM (1996) Discontinuing venom immunotherapy: outcome after five years. J Allergy Clin Immunol 97:579–587
Greter M, Hofmann J, Becher B (2009) Neo-lymphoid aggregates in the adult liver can initiate potent cell-mediated immunity. PLoS Biol 7:e1000109
Grover A, Kim GJ, Lizee G, Tschoi M, Wang G, Wunderlich JR et al (2006) Intralymphatic dendritic cell vaccination induces tumor antigen-specific, skin-homing T lymphocytes. Clin Cancer Res 12:5801–5808
Guidry AJ, O'Brian CN, Oliver SP, Dowlen HH, Douglass LW (1994) Effect of whole *Staphylococcus aureus* and mode of immunization on bovine opsonizing antibodies to capsule. J Dairy Sci 77:2965–2974
Heinzerling L, Basch V, Maloy K, Johansen P, Senti G, Wuthrich B et al (2006) Critical role for DNA vaccination frequency in induction of antigen-specific cytotoxic responses. Vaccine 24:1389–1394
ISAAC (The International Study of Asthma and Allergies in Childhood) Steering Committee (1998) Worldwide variation in prevalence of symptoms of asthma, allergic rhinoconjunctivitis, and atopic eczema: ISAAC. Lancet 351:1225–1232
Johansen P, Haffner AC, Koch F, Zepter K, Erdmann I, Maloy K et al (2005) Direct intralymphatic injection of peptide vaccines enhances immunogenicity. Eur J Immunol 35:568–574
Juillard GJ, Boyer PJ (1977) Intralymphatic immunization: current status. Eur J Cancer 13:439–440
Juillard GJ, Boyer PJ, Snow HD (1976) Intralymphatic infusion of autochthonous tumor cells in canine lymphoma. Int J Radiat Oncol Biol Phys 1:497–503
Juillard GJ, Boyer PJ, Yamashiro CH, Snow HD, Weisenburger TH, McCarthy T et al (1977) Regional intralymphatic infusion (ILI) of irradiated tumor cells with evidence of distant effects. Cancer 39:126–130
Juillard GJ, Boyer PJ, Yamashiro CH (1978) A phase I study of active specific intralymphatic immunotherapy (ASILI). Cancer 41:2215–2225
Juillard GJ, Boyer PJ, Niewisch H, Hom M (1979) Distribution and consequences of cell suspensions following intralymphatic infusion. Bull Cancer 66:217–228
Karrer U, Althage A, Odermatt B, Roberts CW, Korsmeyer SJ, Miyawaki S et al.(1997) On the key role of secondary lymphoid organs in antiviral immune responses studied in alymphoplastic (aly/aly) and spleenless (Hox11$^{-/-}$ mutant mice). J Exp Med 185:2157–2170
Kawabata S, Miller CJ, Lehner T, Fujihashi K, Kubota M, McGhee JR et al (1998) Induction of Th2 cytokine expression for p27-specific IgA B cell responses after targeted lymph node immunization with simian immunodeficiency virus in rhesus macaques. J Infect Dis 177:26–33
Klavinskis LS, Bergmeier LA, Gao L, Mitchell E, Ward RG, Layton G et al (1996) Mucosal or targeted lymph node immunization of macaques with a particulate SIVp27 protein elicits virus-specific CTL in the genito-rectal mucosa and draining lymph nodes. J Immunol 157:2521–2527
Koopman G, Bogers WM, van Gils M, Koornstra W, Barnett S, Morein B et al (2007) Comparison of intranasal with targeted lymph node immunization using PR8-Flu ISCOM adjuvanted HIV antigens in macaques. J Med Virol 79:474–482
Kreiter S, Selmi A, Diken M, Koslowski M, Britten CM, Huber C et al (2010) Intranodal vaccination with naked antigen-encoding RNA elicits potent prophylactic and therapeutic antitumoral immunity. Cancer Res 70:9031–9040

Kundig TM, Bachmann MF, DiPaolo C, Simard JJ, Battegay M, Lother H et al.(1995) Fibroblasts as efficient antigen-presenting cells in lymphoid organs. Science 268:1343–1347

Lehner T, Bergmeier LA, Tao L, Panagiotidi C, Klavinskis LS, Hussain L et al (1994) Targeted lymph node immunization with simian immunodeficiency virus p27 antigen to elicit genital, rectal, and urinary immune responses in nonhuman primates. J Immunol 153:1858–1868

Lehner T, Wang Y, Cranage M, Bergmeier LA, Mitchell E, Tao L et al (1996) Protective mucosal immunity elicited by targeted iliac lymph node immunization with a subunit SIV envelope and core vaccine in macaques. Nat Med 2:767–775

Lehner T, Mitchell E, Bergmeier L, Singh M, Spallek R, Cranage M et al (2000) The role of gammadelta T cells in generating antiviral factors and beta-chemokines in protection against mucosal simian immunodeficiency virus infection. Eur J Immunol 30:2245–2256

Lesimple T, Moisan A, Carsin A, Ollivier I, Mousseau M, Meunier B et al (2003) Injection by various routes of melanoma antigen-associated macrophages: biodistribution and clinical effects. Cancer Immunol Immunother 52:438–444

Lesimple T, Neidhard EM, Vignard V, Lefeuvre C, Adamski H, Labarriere N et al (2006) Immunologic and clinical effects of injecting mature peptide-loaded dendritic cells by intralymphatic and intranodal routes in metastatic melanoma patients. Clin Cancer Res 12:7380–7388

Lockey RF (2001) "ARIA": global guidelines and new forms of allergen immunotherapy. J Allergy Clin Immunol 108:497–499

Lockey RF, Benedict LM, Turkeltaub PC, Bukantz SC (1987) Fatalities from immunotherapy (IT) and skin testing (ST). J Allergy Clin Immunol 79:660–677

Lockey RF, Turkeltaub PC, Olive ES, Hubbard JM, Baird-Warren IA, Bukantz SC (1990) The Hymenoptera venom study. III: safety of venom immunotherapy. J Allergy Clin Immunol 86:775–780

Mackensen A, Krause T, Blum U, Uhrmeister P, Mertelsmann R, Lindemann A (1999) Homing of intravenously and intralymphatically injected human dendritic cells generated in vitro from $CD34^+$ hematopoietic progenitor cells. Cancer Immunol Immunother 48:118–122

Maloy KJ, Erdmann I, Basch V, Sierro S, Kramps TA, Zinkernagel RM et al (2001) Intralymphatic immunization enhances DNA vaccination. Proc Natl Acad Sci USA 98:3299–3303

Manolova V, Flace A, Bauer M, Schwarz K, Saudan P, Bachmann MF (2008) Nanoparticles target distinct dendritic cell populations according to their size. Eur J Immunol 38:1404–1413

Martinez-Gomez JM, Johansen P, Erdmann I, Senti G, Crameri R, Kundig TM (2009a) Intralymphatic injections as a new administration route for allergen-specific immunotherapy. Int Arch Allergy Immunol 150:59–65

Martinez-Gomez JM, Johansen P, Rose H, Steiner M, Senti G, Rhyner C et al (2009b) Targeting the MHC class II pathway of antigen presentation enhances immunogenicity and safety of allergen immunotherapy. Allergy 64:172–178

Moller C, Dreborg S, Ferdousi HA, Halken S, Host A, Jacobsen L et al (2002) Pollen immunotherapy reduces the development of asthma in children with seasonal rhinoconjunctivitis (the PAT-study). J Allergy Clin Immunol 109:251–256

Morse MA, Coleman RE, Akabani G, Niehaus N, Coleman D, Lyerly HK (1999) Migration of human dendritic cells after injection in patients with metastatic malignancies. Cancer Res 59:56–58

Nilsson BO, Svalander PC, Larsson A (1987) Immunization of mice and rabbits by intrasplenic deposition of nanogram quantities of protein attached to Sepharose beads or nitrocellulose paper strips. J Immunol Methods 99:67–75

Norman PS (2004) Immunotherapy: 1999–2004. J Allergy Clin Immunol 113:1013–1023, quiz 24

Ochsenbein AF, Sierro S, Odermatt B, Pericin M, Karrer U, Hermans J et al (2001) Roles of tumour localization, second signals and cross priming in cytotoxic T cell induction. Nature 411:1058–1064

Pajno GB, Barberio G, De Luca F, Morabito L, Parmiani S (2001) Prevention of new sensitizations in asthmatic children monosensitized to house dust mite by specific immunotherapy. A six-year follow-up study. Clin Exp Allergy 31:1392–1397

Pierson-Mullany LK, Jackola D, Blumenthal M, Rosenberg A (2000) Altered allergen binding capacities of Amb a 1-specific IgE and IgG4 from ragweed-sensitive patients receiving immunotherapy. Ann Allergy Asthma Immunol 84:241–243

Quillien V, Moisan A, Carsin A, Lesimple T, Lefeuvre C, Adamski H et al (2005) Biodistribution of radiolabelled human dendritic cells injected by various routes. Eur J Nucl Med Mol Imaging 32:731–741

Rhyner C, Kundig T, Akdis CA, Crameri R (2007) Targeting the MHC II presentation pathway in allergy vaccine development. Biochem Soc Trans 35:833–834

Senti G, Prinz Vavricka BM, Erdmann I, Diaz MI, Markus R, McCormack SJ et al (2008) Intralymphatic allergen administration renders specific immunotherapy faster and safer: a randomized controlled trial. Proc Natl Acad Sci USA 105:17908–17912

Sigel MB, Sinha YN, VanderLaan WP (1983) Production of antibodies by inoculation into lymph nodes. Methods Enzymol 93:3–12

Smith KA, Tam VL, Wong RM, Pagarigan RR, Meisenburg BL, Joea DK et al (2009) Enhancing DNA vaccination by sequential injection of lymph nodes with plasmid vectors and peptides. Vaccine 27:2603–2615

Stewart GE, II, Lockey RF (1992) Systemic reactions from allergen immunotherapy. J Allergy Clin Immunol 90:567–578

Storni T, Ruedl C, Schwarz K, Schwendener RA, Renner WA, Bachmann MF (2004) Nonmethylated CG motifs packaged into virus-like particles induce protective cytotoxic T cell responses in the absence of systemic side effects. J Immunol 172:1777–1785

Tagawa ST, Lee P, Snively J, Boswell W, Ounpraseuth S, Lee S et al (2003) Phase I study of intranodal delivery of a plasmid DNA vaccine for patients with Stage IV melanoma. Cancer 98:144–154

Thomas R, Chambers M, Boytar R, Barker K, Cavanagh LL, MacFadyen S et al (1999) Immature human monocyte-derived dendritic cells migrate rapidly to draining lymph nodes after intradermal injection for melanoma immunotherapy. Melanoma Res 9:474–481

Till SJ, Francis JN, Nouri-Aria K, Durham SR (2004) Mechanisms of immunotherapy. J Allergy Clin Immunol 113:1025–1034, quiz 35

Varney VA, Gaga M, Frew AJ, Aber VR, Kay AB, Durham SR (1991) Usefulness of immunotherapy in patients with severe summer hay fever uncontrolled by antiallergic drugs. Bmj 302:265–269

Verlato G, Corsico A, Villani S, Cerveri I, Migliore E, Accordini S et al (2003) Is the prevalence of adult asthma and allergic rhinitis still increasing? Results of an Italian study. J Allergy Clin Immunol 111:1232–1238

Vissers JL, van Esch BC, Hofman GA, Kapsenberg ML, Weller FR, van Oosterhout AJ (2004) Allergen immunotherapy induces a suppressive memory response mediated by IL-10 in a mouse asthma model. J Allergy Clin Immunol 113:1204–1210

von Beust BR, Johansen P, Smith KA, Bot A, Storni T, Kundig TM (2005) Improving the therapeutic index of CpG oligodeoxynucleotides by intralymphatic administration. Eur J Immunol 35:1869–1876

Weber J, Boswell W, Smith J, Hersh E, Snively J, Diaz M et al (2008) Phase 1 trial of intranodal injection of a Melan-A/MART-1 DNA plasmid vaccine in patients with stage IV melanoma. J Immunother 31:215–223

Wuthrich B, Schindler C, Medici TC, Zellweger JP, Leuenberger P (1996) IgE levels, atopy markers and hay fever in relation to age, sex and smoking status in a normal adult Swiss population. SAPALDIA (Swiss study on air pollution and lung diseases in adults) Team. Int Arch Allergy Immunol 111:396–402

Zinkernagel RM (2000) Localization dose and time of antigens determine immune reactivity. Semin Immunol 12:163–171, discussion 257–344

Zinkernagel RM, Ehl S, Aichele P, Oehen S, Kundig T, Hengartner H (1997) Antigen localisation regulates immune responses in a dose- and time-dependent fashion: a geographical view of immune reactivity. Immunol Rev 156:199–209

Induction of Allergen-Specific Tolerance via Mucosal Routes

Laurent Mascarell, Aline Zimmer, Laurence Van Overtvelt, Sophie Tourdot and Philippe Moingeon

Abstract Allergen-specific immunotherapy is the only curative treatment of allergies against insect venom, house dust mites, tree/grass pollens, or cat dander. Subcutaneous immunotherapy is successful to reorient the immune system and re-establish long-term tolerance. However, major drawbacks for using this route include: repeated injections, as well as the risk of anaphylaxis. In this context, alternative mucosal routes of administration are being considered together with the combined use of adjuvants/vector systems and recombinant allergens or peptide fragments. Herein, we review the current status in the use of mucosal routes (i.e., sublingual, oral, intranasal) for allergen-specific immunotherapy, as well as the latest understanding with respect to underlying mechanisms of action.

L. Mascarell · A. Zimmer · L. Van Overtvelt · S. Tourdot · P. Moingeon (✉)
Research and Development, Stallergènes, 6 rue Alexis de Tocqueville, 92160 Antony, France
e-mail: pmoingeon@stallergenes.fr

L. Mascarell
e-mail: lmascarell@stallergenes.fr

A. Zimmer
e-mail: azimmer@stallergenes.fr

L. Van Overtvelt
e-mail: lvanovertvelt@stallergenes.fr

S. Tourdot
e-mail: stourdot@stallergenes.fr

Current Topics in Microbiology and Immunology (2011) 352: 85–105
DOI: 10.1007/82_2011_132

Published Online: 12 May 2011

Contents

1 Introduction

The first successful studies of allergen-immunotherapy were conducted in patients with hay fever in 1911, by Noon et al. As of today, many double blind, placebo-controlled (DBPC) studies have shown that subcutaneous allergen-specific immunotherapy (SCIT) is effective in decreasing both immediate and late-phase symptoms as well as the need for medication, when applied to a variety of type I allergies involving either insect venom, house dust mites, grass and tree pollens, or animal epithelia (Bousquet et al. 1998; Larche 2000; Gehlhar et al. 1999; Michils et al. 1998; Pichler and Pichler 2001; Moller et al. 2002; Powell et al. 2007). In terms of mechanisms, successful SCIT is often associated with a decrease in seric allergen-specific IgE antibodies together with an increase in IgG4, including potential blocking antibodies (Wachholz 2003; Pierson-Mullany et al. 2000). Successful SCIT redirects allergen-specific Th2 $CD4^+$ cells (producing IL4, IL5, and IL13) (Durham and Till 1998; El Biaze et al. 2003) toward the Th1 type (secreting IL12/IFNγ) (Mavroleon 1998; Hamid et al. 1997; Benjaponpitak et al. 1999; Ebner et al. 1997; Secrist et al. 1993). In addition, SCIT promotes allergen-specific $CD4^+$ regulatory T cells (i.e., IL10-producing Tr1 or $CD4^+CD25^+$ cells) (Robinson et al. 2004; Meiler et al. 2008). Several drawbacks currently limit the application of SCIT. First of all, repeated injections make this treatment cumbersome, most particularly for children. In addition, systemic reactions to SCIT, albeit infrequent, may occur, which include anaphylactic shocks (Medicines 1986). In this context, tolerance induction via non-invasive mucosal routes has raised considerable interest over the last two decades. Also, various non-mutually exclusive immune mechanisms have been discovered including (i) the development of active suppression via regulatory T cells, (ii) the inhibition of inappropriate immune responses through cellular anergy or clonal deletion, (iii) the generation of blocking antibodies (Faria and Weiner 2005, 2006a, b).

Herein, we review the pertinence of various mucosal routes (i.e., nasal, oral, and sublingual) of allergen administration as alternatives to SCIT. Out of these mucosal routes, only the sublingual one has clearly been documented as efficacious for establishing antigen-specific tolerance in humans, in the context of large double blind placebo-controlled (DBPC) clinical studies conducted both in adults and children. Immune mechanisms associated with successful specific mucosal immunotherapy are discussed in the context of new strategies based on vectors/adjuvant molecules in order to better target antigen-presenting cells with tolerogenic capacity.

2 Tolerance Induction by Mucosal Immunotherapy

2.1 General Comments

Increasing evidence suggests that dendritic cells (DCs) play a crucial role in the regulation of mucosal immunity and tolerance, as a consequence of their capacity to direct the fate of T cells. The physiology of mucosal APCs, most particularly their capacity to support the differentiation of regulatory T cells, likely explains why the default response is usually tolerogenic at mucosal surfaces. The level of costimulatory molecules as well as the cytokine milieu influence the degree of antigen-presenting cell (APC) maturation and activation, leading to systemic or suppressive T cell responses (MacPherson et al. 2004). In most circumstances, mature DCs (mDCs) trigger specific effector T cells, whereas immature or semi-mature DCs (iDCs or smDCs) rather induce regulatory T cells, clonal deletion or hypo responsiveness (Steinman et al. 2003; Hawiger et al. 2001). Most particularly, iDCs continuously capture, transport, and present self-antigens as well as micro-environmental proteins from mucosal tissues to lymphoid organs to maintain tolerance (Pugh et al. 1983; Liu et al. 1998; Huang et al. 2000). Recent studies suggest that IL10-producing iDCs prime immunological tolerance through $Tr1^+$ regulatory T cells in both mice and humans (Jonuleit et al. 2000; Menges et al. 2002).

APCs from the lamina propria of the small intestine, including $CD11b^+$ $CD11c^+$ DCs and $CD11b^+$ $F4/80^+$ $CD11c^-$ macrophages, promote the development of extrathymic $Foxp3^+$ Treg due to the presence of TGFβ and retinoic acid (RA), i.e., a vitamin A metabolite highly expressed in gut-associated lymphoid tissue (GALT) (Sun et al. 2007; Denning et al. 2007). Together, these data demonstrate that the intestinal immune system has evolved to promote tolerance over inflammation. Although the oral immune system is prone as well to induce specific tolerance (Iwasaki and Kelsall 1999; Mascarell et al. 2008; Sun et al. 2008), it also comprises local effector mechanisms in the form of resident mucosal $CD4^+$ T cells able to promote Th1, Th2 and Th17 patterns of polarization upon polyclonal activation (Mascarell et al. 2009). In agreement with these observations, recent data further demonstrate that the oral immune system retains the capacity to promote protective Th1 effector responses in draining lymph nodes (Cuburu et al. 2007; Song et al. 2008), and that IL17 producing $CD4^+$ T cells are found within the oral cavity (Conti et al. 2009).

2.2 Intranasal Immunotherapy

Biodistribution studies in humans of radiolabeled *Parietaria judaica* allergen (Par j 1) following intranasal administration suggest that the allergen quickly disappears from the nasal cavity, is transported to the pharynx, and then absorbed through the gastrointestinal tract, reaching a plasmatic peak between 1.5 and 3 h after administration (Bagnasco et al. 1997; Passalacqua et al. 2005). Interestingly, nasal clearance is superior in allergic patients when compared to healthy volunteers, suggesting an IgE-mediated capture mechanism in Par j 1 sensitized patients.

Local nasal immunotherapy (LNIT) has been explored during the last three decades, with some encouraging results, both in terms of safety and efficacy in patients with allergic rhinitis (Canonica and Passalacqua 2003) (Table 1). Pioneer studies using either natural biological or chemically-modified (allergoid) forms demonstrated a significant reduction in both symptoms and requirement for symptomatic medication in patients allergic to ragweed and grass pollens (Deuschl and Johansson 1977; Nickelsen et al. 1981a, b; Georgitis et al. 1983). However, no cumulative effect of LNIT could be confirmed, since the administration of allergoid grass extracts was ineffective in the second year of treatment (Nickelsen et al. 1983). In addition, macronized powder forms of pollens (e.g., parietaria, birch, and grass) or mites as well as strips coated with mite extracts have been used in LNIT and shown to improve clinical efficacy, while reducing local side effects in patients with rhinitis (Andri et al. 1992, 1993, 1996; D'Amato et al. 1995; Andri and Senna 1995; Bellussi et al. 2002; Tsai et al. 2009). Some clinical studies suggested a long lasting protective effect (i.e., up to three or four years after the end of the treatment), most particularly on nasal symptoms (Passalacqua et al. 1997; Andri and Falagiani 2003). Adverse effects were rarely observed (Georgitis et al. 1983) and were limited to the upper respiratory tract (Andri et al. 1992).

Regarding immunological changes associated in humans with LNIT, some studies have shown an increase in serum or nasal IgE, IgG, and IgA antibodies, (Deuschl and Johansson 1977; Georgitis et al. 1983; Nickelsen et al. 1981a, b) whereas others failed to detect any differences in antibody responses (D'Amato et al. 1995). Locally, a reduction of inflammatory cellular infiltrates together with a decrease in histamine and eosinophil cationic protein (ECP) levels in nasal secretions have been observed (Passalacqua et al. 1997; Andri and Falagiani 2003).

To further decipher immune mechanisms associated with intranasal immunotherapy, murine models of established asthma have been developed using prophylactic or therapeutic intranasal treatment with either allergen extracts (from pollen or mite), purified/recombinant major allergens (Bet v 1, Der p 1) or polypeptide fragments (Bet v 1, Phl p 1, and Phl p 5) alone or together with an adjuvant (CpG-ODN, Flagelin, fungal immunomodulatory protein) or a vector system such as probiotics (e.g., *Lactobacillus plantarum*). In those pre-clinical models, LNIT reduced both airway hyperresponsiveness (AHR), cellular infiltration in lungs, specific seric IgE, the IgG1/IgG2a antibody ratio, and IL5 production in T cells.

Table 1 Comparative properties of mucosal immunization routes

Route of immunization	Allergens	Comments	References
Local nasal immunotherapy (LNIT)	Pollens (ragweed, grasses, parietaria, birch), house dust mites	Clinical efficacy: Local nasal immunotherapy (LNIT) is safe and induces a reduction in both symptoms and medication scores in patients with allergic rhinitis to house dust mite (HDM) and pollens (tree and grass). Chemically modified allergens (allergoids) are better-tolerated than aqueous extracts, but the therapeutic benefit is decreased. Some studies demonstrate a long lasting protective effect on nasal symptoms (grass allergy; three to four years after the end of the treatment). Nevertheless, LNIT requires technical skills to control the dose administered, thus impeding its large utilization in allergen-specific immunotherapy	Canonica and Passalacqua (2003); Deuschl and Johansson (1977); Nickelsen et al. (1981a, b, 1983); Georgitis et al. (1983); Andri et al. (1992, 1993, 1996); D'Amato et al. (1995); Andri and Senna (1995); Bellussi et al. (2002); Tsai et al. (2009); Passalacqua et al. (1997); Andri and Falagiani (2003)
	Used as: natural extracts, allergoids, macronized powder forms, strips coated extracts	Immune mechanisms: *Antibody responses*: LNIT with aqueous extracts or allergoids (ragweed and grass) is associated with an increase in seric or nasal allergen-specific IgA, IgE, and IgG antibodies.	Deuschl and Johansson (1977); Georgitis et al. (1983); D'Amato et al. (1995); Nickelsen et al. (1981a, b)
		Cellular responses: Successful LNIT to parietaria significantly reduces cellular infiltration as well as histamine and eosinophil cationic protein (ECP) nasal secretion	Passalacqua et al. (1997); Andri and Falagiani (2003)
		Pre-clinical models and candidate vaccines: In murine models of established asthma, prophylactic or therapeutic intranasal treatments with either allergen extracts (pollen, mite), purified/recombinant major allergen (i.e., Bet v 1, Der p 1) or polypeptide fragments (i.e., rBet v 1, rPhl p 1, and rPhl p 5) alone or together with an immunopotentiator (CpG-ODN, Flagelin, fungal immunomodulatory protein, *Lactobacillus plantarum*) decrease the Th2 polarization (i.e., reduced AHR, cellular infiltration, seric IgE, IgG1/IgG2a ratio, and IL5 production) together with an increased expression of IgA in saliva or TGFβ, IL10, and Foxp3 in $CD4^+$ T cells	Liu and Tsai (2005); Daniel et al. (2006); Hisbergues et al. (2007); Robinson et al. (2004); Lee et al. (2008); Hufnagl et al. (2008); Winkler et al. (2006)

(continued)

Table 1 (continued)

Route of immunization	Allergens	Comments	References
Oral immunotherapy (OIT)	Pollens (ragweed, grasses, artemisia, birch), house dust mites, food allergens (milk, egg), autoimmune disease related antigen (type I diabetes, multiple sclerosis, rheumatoid arthritis, uveitis, and thyroiditis)	Clinical efficacy: Grass pollen OIT (low or high doses) is ineffective in terms of therapeutic effects, whereas OIT with birch, ragweed, artemisia pollens or HDM extracts (high doses) reduces asthma/rhinitis symptoms both in adults and children	Rebien et al. (1982); Taudorf and Weeke (1983); Mosbech et al. (1987); Urbanek et al. (1990); Taudorf et al. (1987, 1989); Moller et al. (1986); Leng et al. (1990); Litwin et al. (1997); Giovane et al. (1994); Meglio et al. (2004, 2008)
		In OIT with food allergen, children received increasing doses of milk or egg which re-install tolerance toward the allergens in most cases. One placebo-controlled study of OIT for cow's milk and egg allergies does not report an enhanced tolerance recovery. A major drawback of those studies is that they report outcomes in small cohorts of patients often lacking a control group to analyze spontaneous improvement	Buchanan et al. (2007); Staden et al. (2007); Longo et al. (2008)
		OIT for autoimmune diseases has been tested in humans using antigenic peptides or purified/recombinant proteins but failed to demonstrate significant effects over the placebo group	Faria and Weiner (2006)
	Used as: natural extract in aqueous, freeze-dried, powder forms, enterosoluble capsules	Immune mechanisms: *Antibody responses*: OIT with grass pollen allergen extracts does not alter humoral (IgE, IgG) responses. OIT with birch, ragweed, artemisia pollens, or mites extracts decreases seric IgE and up-regulates seric IgG1/IgG4 antibodies in allergic patients (adults and children)	Rebien et al. (1982); Taudorf and Weeke (1983); Taudorf et al. (1987); Moller et al. (1986); Taudorf et al. (1989); Leng et al. (1990); Litwin et al. (1997); Giovane et al. (1994)
		Successful OIT as well as spontaneous re-establishment of oral tolerance to cow's milk or egg allergens are associated with an increase in specific IgG4 and a reduction of food-specific IgE antibody levels	Burks et al. (2008); Staden et al. (2007); Longo et al. (2008); Patriarca et al. (2003); Skripak et al. (2008)

(continued)

Table 1 (continued)

Route of immunization	Allergens	Comments	References
		Cellular responses: No changes in histamine secretion by basophils following OIT with grass pollen allergen extracts. In the absence of clinical effect, TGFβ-producing Th3 regulatory cells were induced in patients treated for diabetes or multiple sclerosis	Faria and Weiner (2006); Taudorf and Weeke (1983)
		Pre-clinical models and candidate vaccines: Experimental animal models of autoimmune diseases show that $CD4^+$ regulatory T cells involved in oral tolerance induction are highly heterogeneous and include Th3 cells (producing TGFβ and/or IL10), Tr1 cells (producing IL10) and $CD4^+$ $CD25^+$ cells secreting TGFβ or mediating their suppressive function through CTLA-4, PD-1, or latency-associated peptide (LAP) molecules. For example, oral administration of antigen coupled with non toxic cholera toxin B subunit (CTB) as a mucosal adjuvant promotes peripheral tolerance induction through the induction of both $CD4^+$ $CD25^+$ $Foxp3^+$ and $CD4^+$ $Foxp3^-$ LAP^+ TGFβ^+ regulatory T cells	Faria and Weiner (2006); Sun et al. (2008); Nakamura et al. (2001); Oida et al. (2003); Chen et al. (2008)
Sublingual immunotherapy (SLIT)	Venoms, pollens (ragweed, birch, grasses, parietaria, olive), house dust mites	Clinical efficacy: SLIT is efficient in treating type I allergies to either house dust mites or pollens (from grass, parietaria, olive, ragweed, cupressus). It reduces both symptoms and medication requirements in adults and children. SLIT exhibits a favorable safety profile and long lasting effects in adults and children with rhinitis. SLIT using grass pollen or HDM sublingual tablets has shown a significant reduction in rhinitis symptoms together with an excellent safety profile in the context of large scale placebo-controlled phase III studies	Wilson et al. (2003); Khinchi et al. (2004); Wilson et al. (2005); Olaguibel and Alvarez Puebla (2005); Calamita et al. (2006); Penagos et al. (2006); Larenas-Linnemann (2009); Passalacqua et al. (2004); Pajno et al. (2003); Mascarell et al. (2006); Antunez et al. (2008); Baena-Cagnani et al. (2005); Fiocchi et al. (2005); Didier et al. (2006); Dahl et al. (2006); Ibanez et al. (2007); Dahl et al. (2008); Wahn et al. (2009); Didier et al. (2009); Horak et al. (2009); Malling et al. (2009)

(continued)

Table 1 (continued)

Route of immunization	Allergens	Comments	References
	Used as: natural biological extracts, allergoids, tablets	Immune mechanisms: *Antibody responses*: SLIT enhances allergen-specific IgG4 antibodies while decreasing IgE antibodies. In some studies, allergen-specific IgA antibodies are induced	Mascarell et al. (2006); Bahceciler et al. (2005)
		Cellular responses: SLIT to grass pollen or HDM decreases ECP and tryptase nasal secretion. In some studies SLIT used against house dust mites, birch, and grass pollens elicit both Th1 and regulatory T cells (i.e., IL10-producing Tr1 or Foxp3$^+$ CD4$^+$ CD25$^+$ cells) in peripheral blood or in the nasal mucosa	Meiler et al. (2008); Marcucci et al. (2001, 2003); Passalacqua et al. (1998); Jutel et al. (2003); Gardner et al. (2004); Taylor et al. (2004); Ciprandi et al. (2005); Bohle et al. (2007); Radulovic et al. (2008); Cosmi et al. (2006)
		Pre-clinical models and candidate vaccines: The lingual immune system is prone to induce specific tolerance since mucosal APCs including plasmacytoïd, CD11b$^+$CD11c$^+$ and CD11b$^+$ CD11c$^-$ DCs as well as Langerhans cells promote Th1/Treg responses in draining lymph nodes. Targeting lingual APCs with adjuvants (i.e., selected strains of Lactobacilli, Pam3CSK4, OM-294-BA-MP as well as immunosuppressive drugs e.g., glucocorticoids plus vitamin D3) or with mucoadhesive particles (polysaccharidic core nanoparticles (PSC) or chitosan) as vector systems improve SLIT efficacy in a therapeutic murine model of asthma by inhibiting Th2 responses (reduction of AHR, lung inflammation, eosinophils in bronchoalveolar lavages, IL5, and IL13 production) while inducing IFNγ (Th1) and/or IL10 (Treg) producing T cells. In humans, the Th1 adjuvant monophosphoryl lipid A (MPL) is currently under investigation in sublingual immunotherapy	Mascarell et al. (2007, 2008); Allam et al. (2003, 2008a); Van Overtvelt et al. (2008); Lombardi et al. (2008); Razafindratsita et al. (2007); Saint-Lu et al. (2009)

It also increased allergen-specific IgA in saliva and elicited IFNγ and IL10 production by circulating CD4$^+$ T cells (Liu and Tsai 2005; Daniel et al. 2006; Hisbergues et al. 2007; Mousavi et al. 2008; Lee et al. 2008; Hufnagl et al. 2008). In a murine model of birch pollen allergy, immunological tolerance to Bet v 1 correlated with an increased expression of both transforming growth factor-beta (TGFβ), and IL10, as well as the induction of Foxp3$^+$ CD4$^+$ T cells, thus highlighting an active regulatory mechanism (Winkler et al. 2006).

Altogether, LNIT appears safe and efficient in treating allergic rhinitis linked with pollen and mite. As of today, however, LNIT efficacy has not yet been documented in the context of large clinical studies versus placebo. Also, nasal application of allergen extracts makes it difficult to control the exact dose administered to patients, thus currently limiting its broad use in allergen-specific immunotherapy.

2.3 Oral Immunotherapy

In the 1980s, oral immunotherapy (OIT) has been studied in both adults and children with pollen-induced allergic rhinitis (Rebien et al. 1982; Taudorf and Weeke 1983; Mosbech et al. 1987; Urbanek et al. 1990; Taudorf et al. 1987, 1989; Moller et al. 1986; Leng et al. 1990; Litwin et al. 1997) (Table 1). A number of these studies were performed with grass pollen allergens presented either as an aqueous solution, or as powder or enterosoluble forms (Rebien et al. 1982; Taudorf and Weeke 1983; Mosbech et al. 1987; Urbanek et al. 1990). Although OIT with grass pollen was well-tolerated, it has been shown to be clinically ineffective. In addition, no significant changes in seric allergen-specific IgG or IgE levels were detected in comparison to placebo (Rebien et al. 1982; Taudorf and Weeke 1983). Conversely, OIT with high doses of selected allergen aqueous extracts (e.g., *Dermatophagoides pteronyssinus or Artemisia*) (Leng et al. 1990; Giovane et al. 1994) or using encapsulated allergens (e.g., birch or ragweed pollens) (Taudorf et al. 1987, 1989; Moller et al. 1986; Litwin et al. 1997) showed evidence of safety and efficacy associated with a significant decrease in serum-specific IgE antibodies, and an upregulation of serum-specific IgG1/IgG4 antibody levels in allergic patients (adults and children).

OIT is currently being evaluated to re-establish the tolerance to dietary proteins in children who have developed food allergies, such as cow's milk and egg allergies (Burks et al. 2008). Several clinical studies have been conducted in children failing to outgrown those allergies with food allergens (Meglio et al. 2004, 2008; Buchanan et al. 2007; Staden et al. 2007; Longo et al. 2008). Due to the risk of severe reactions, desensitization protocols rely upon the administration of small incremental doses of the food allergen in order to reach amounts normally tolerated (from micrograms to milligrams to grams) followed by a food challenge at the end of the study protocol to evaluate efficacy. In a standardized OIT protocol applied to cow's milk allergy, desensitization was totally or partially successful in

85% of cases with an acceptable safety profile (Meglio et al. 2004). In addition, a long lasting efficacy was observed for up to 4–5 years after the end of treatment (Meglio et al. 2008). Also, encouraging results were obtained in egg OIT (Buchanan et al. 2007). One limitation of those studies is that they rely upon small cohorts of patients, they often lack a control group and do not measure spontaneous outgrowth. For example, a randomized, placebo-controlled study of OIT for cow's milk and egg allergies comparing a control group (with allergen eviction) with the tolerance induction group, concluded that both groups exhibited tolerance to allergens, thus, pointing out that OIT for food allergy should take into consideration the spontaneous rate of recovery of patients (Staden et al. 2007). Nonetheless, a recent study of children with a severe allergy to cow's milk showed a significant 90% increase in tolerated milk intake, only in the group receiving the therapy, whereas the eviction control group failed the food challenge after 1 year (Longo et al. 2008). These studies raise questions regarding criteria for patient selection, dose incrementation, and treatment duration.

In terms of serological changes, OIT for cow's milk leads to a significant decrease in food-specific IgE levels (Longo et al. 2008; Patriarca et al. 2003) concomitantly with an increase in specific IgG4 levels (Longo et al. 2008; Patriarca et al. 2003; Skripak et al. 2008). In the case of spontaneous re-establishment of oral tolerance to cow's milk or egg allergens in children, allergen-specific IgE levels also decrease significantly (Staden et al. 2007). Accordingly, children whose allergy resolves spontaneously exhibit a reorientation of preexisting Th2 responses toward Th1 and regulatory T cells (Burks et al. 2008).

Oral tolerance has been further tested in human autoimmune diseases such as type I diabetes, multiple sclerosis, rheumatoid arthritis, uveitis and thyroiditis, using antigenic peptides as well as purified or recombinant proteins (Faria and Weiner 2006a). Although the induction of regulatory mechanisms such as TGFβ-producing Th3 cells was observed in patients treated for diabetes or multiple sclerosis, phase II/III trials showed no significant effect over the placebo group (Faria and Weiner 2006b). In contrast, specific oral tolerance regimens have demonstrated promising results in experimental animal models of autoimmune diseases. In those experiments, high doses of antigen administered orally promote T cell depletion or anergy (Faria and Weiner 2005), whereas low doses rather induce suppressive mechanisms involving regulatory T cells. Such regulatory T cells are highly heterogeneous and include Th3 cells (producing TGFβ and/or IL10), Tr1 cells (producing IL10), and $CD4^+$ $CD25^+$ T cells mediating their suppressive function through cytokine secretion, or cell contact-dependent mechanisms involving the CTLA-4 or PD-1 molecules (Faria and Weiner 2006a). In addition, new subsets ($CD4^+$ $CD25^-$ or $CD4^+$ $CD25^+$) of regulatory T cells have been described which express latency-associated peptide (LAP), secrete TGFβ and corresponding surface receptors at the cell surface, thus mediating regulatory functions through both soluble factors and cell contact (Nakamura et al. 2001; Oida et al. 2003; Chen et al. 2008).

Altogether, although oral tolerance induction has been successful in a number of animal models, the clinical efficacy of OIT remains to be firmly established in humans.

The inability of the protein to bypass the gastrointestinal barrier remains problematic in the oral administration of protein drugs. In order to overcome problems of low allergen/protein bioavailability and absorption after OIT, current investigations are focusing on novel and enhanced delivery systems for a safe oral administration of the antigen.

2.4 Sublingual Immunotherapy

Allergen-specific sublingual immunotherapy (SLIT) has been investigated in allergic patients since 1984 (Bousquet et al. 1999; La Rosa et al. 1999; Wilson et al. 2003; Clavel et al. 1998; Vourdas et al. 1998; Bousquet et al. 2001; Pajno et al. 2000; Marogna et al. 2005) (Table 1). During SLIT, the allergen extract is applied as a solution or as a tablet and kept under the tongue for at least 1–2 min, thus facilitating allergen capture by oral Langerhans cells (oLCs). As of today, more than one billion doses have been administered to humans with an excellent safety profile, demonstrating that SLIT is a valid alternative to SCIT (Khinchi et al. 2004). SLIT is efficient in treating type I allergies to either house dust mites, pollens (from grass, parietaria, olive, ragweed, cupressus) or cat dander in adults and children, with a reduction of both symptoms and medication requirements. As such, SLIT can be used in patients with rhinitis with or without mild-asthma (Wilson et al. 2003, 2005; Olaguibel and Alvarez Puebla 2005; Calamita et al. 2006; Penagos et al. 2006; Larenas-Linnemann 2009; Passalacqua et al. 2004; Pajno et al. 2003; Mascarell et al. 2006). Comparative clinical trials in birch pollen-allergic adults or mite-allergic children revealed no statistical difference in terms of efficacy between SCIT and SLIT when high-dose SLIT regimens were used (Khinchi et al. 2004; Antunez et al. 2008). Also, long-term clinical benefits are observed following SLIT in adults and children with rhinitis (Wilson et al. 2003). The safety and efficacy profile of high-dose immunotherapy has been confirmed in children younger than 5 years (Baena-Cagnani et al. 2005; Fiocchi et al. 2005). As of today, the pertinence of SLIT for tolerance induction in humans has been definitively established by multiple DBPC phase III studies conducted in large cohorts of patients allergic to grass pollen (Didier et al. 2006, 2009; Dahl et al. 2006, 2008; Ibanez et al. 2007; Wahn et al. 2009; Horak et al. 2009; Malling et al. 2009). In addition, house dust mite sublingual tablets tested in 509 adults patients in a pivotal phase IIb/III clinical trial induced a significant decrease in rhinitis symptoms while demonstrating a good safety profile after only 1 year of treatment (our unpublished data).

Similarly to SCIT, SLIT reduces allergen-specific inflammatory responses at various levels. For example, it decreases ECP and tryptase nasal secretion (Marcucci et al. 2001, 2003; Passalacqua et al. 1998). It also enhances specific seric IgG4 while decreasing IgE antibodies (Mascarell et al. 2006; Bahceciler et al. 2005), thus inhibiting basophil or mast cell (MC) degranulation. SLIT elicits both Th1 and regulatory T cells (i.e., IL10-producing Tr1 or Foxp3^{+} CD4^{+} CD25^{+} T cells) in peripheral blood or in the nasal mucosa (Meiler et al. 2008; Jutel et al. 2003; Gardner et al. 2004; Taylor et al. 2004; Ciprandi et al. 2005; Bohle et al. 2007; Radulovic et al. 2008; Cosmi et al. 2006).

APCs identified thus far in the lingual oral mucosa of both mice and humans, consist of oLCs, myeloid $CD11b^+$ $CD11c^-$, $CD11b^+$ $CD11c^+$ as well as plasmacytoid DCs (Mascarell et al. 2008; Allam et al. 2003) with a semi-mature phenotype ($CD40^-$ $CD80^-$ $CD86^+$), consistent with a tolerogenic function (Steinman et al. 2003; Hawiger et al. 2001). Those oral APCs located at the mucosal/submucosal junction are likely involved in antigen capture during SLIT (Mascarell et al. 2008) and represent a privileged target for tolerance induction, since they induce IFNγ and/or IL10 producing $CD4^+$ T cells mediating suppressive functions (Mascarell et al. 2008; Allam et al. 2008a). Also, cross-linking of high affinity receptors for IgE (FcεRI) on human oLCs induces regulatory molecules such as TGFβ, IL10, or indoleamine 2,3-dioxygenase (IDO) (Allam et al. 2003; Novak et al. 2001). In contrast, pro-inflammatory cells, i.e., MCs and eosinophils, are located in submucosal tissues in humans and mice (Marcucci et al. 2007; Allam et al. 2008a), suggesting that allergen contact with such cells might be limited during SLIT. Differences in distribution of oLCs and MCs have been observed within the oral cavity, with the vestibular region identified as the most favorable site for allergen application during sublingual immunotherapy, given its high oLCs and low MCs density (Allam et al. 2008b). In mice, resident mucosal $CD4^+$ T cells co-localize with $CD11b^+$ tolerogenic APCs in the lamina propria, suggesting that the lingual immune system is organized in a similar manner to the small intestine, another critical site for tolerance induction (Denning et al. 2007; Mascarell et al. 2008). Resident mucosal $CD4^+$ T cells express the mucosal homing receptor $\alpha E\beta 7$ integrin CD103, also described as a regulatory marker (Suffia et al. 2005; Allakhverdi et al. 2006).

3 Interest in Adjuvants and Vector Systems for Mucosal Immunization

Given the dual capacity of mucosal immune systems, appropriate signalling to APCs e.g., with immunopotentiators (i.e., synthetic or biological adjuvant molecules) or enhanced targeting via vector systems are needed to promote tolerance over inflammation. For example, selected strains of Lactobacilli have been shown to enhance SLIT efficacy in a therapeutic murine model of asthma (Van Overtvelt et al. 2008). Triggering Toll like receptors (TLR) by lipid A derivatives or lipopeptides (Pam3CSK4 and OM-294-BA-MP, respectively) as well as immunosuppressive drugs (e.g., glucocorticoids with vitamin D3) are also effective in improving SLIT efficacy (Van Overtvelt et al. 2008; Mascarell et al. 2007; Lombardi et al. 2008). In allergen-specific immunotherapy, the use of Th1 adjuvants to potentiate tolerance induction is also currently under investigation. Cytosine-guanine oligonucleotides (CpG) (Simons et al. 2004) and monophosphoryl lipid A (MPL)

(Drachenberg et al. 2001, 2003) have been shown to be effective in ragweed and grass pollen subcutaneous immunotherapy, respectively. The latter is also presently being tested in sublingual immunotherapy regimens in humans.

Selected formulations can be used to present allergens in a particulate form, thereby targeting APCs with a phagocytic property. For example, targeting oral APCs following sublingual administration of OVA formulated within mucoadhesive particles (e.g., polysaccharidic core nanoparticles or chitosan) induces the proliferation of antigen specific suppressive T cells producing IFNγ/IL10 in draining cervical lymph nodes. Sublingual administration of OVA formulated with such particules enhances tolerance induction in mice with established asthma, with a dramatic reduction of both AHR, lung inflammation, eosinophils numbers in bronchoalveolar lavages, as well as antigen-specific Th2 responses (Razafindratsita et al. 2007; Saint-Lu et al. 2009). Other delivery systems targeting DCs are currently being considered (Bohle et al. 2004; El Azami El Idrissi et al. 2002; Jeannin et al. 2000; Goetsch et al. 2001; Haicheur et al. 2003; Bonifaz et al. 2004; Santeliz et al. 2002; Tighe et al. 2000). For instance, the adenylate cyclase (CyaA) from Bordetella pertussis (El Azami El Idrissi et al. 2002), the B subunit of shiga toxin (STxB) (Haicheur et al. 2003), the outer membrane protein A from *Klebsiella pneumoniae* (kpOmpA) (Jeannin et al. 2000; Goetsch et al. 2001) or the bacterial cell surface protein of *Geobacillus stearothermophilus* (S-layer) (Bohle et al. 2004) target DCs and prime efficient Th1 cellular responses. Also, anti-DEC-205 antibodies coupled with antigen target DCs, and induce strong T cell responses in mice when administered together with anti-CD40 antibodies (Bonifaz et al. 2004). Whether or not such delivery systems are relevant to induce allergen-specific tolerance by mucosal routes remain to be addressed.

4 Conclusions

The development of second generation mucosal based-vaccines will benefit from a better understanding of mucosal immune systems. The latter comprise various subsets of tolerogenic APCs organized in a compartmentalized manner and programmed to induce Th1/Treg responses. Based on placebo-controlled clinical studies conducted in large cohort of patients, the sublingual route is as of today the only firmly proven mucosal route to establish tolerance in humans. Targeting the allergen to tolerogenic mucosal DCs using vector systems, mucoadhesive particulate formulations or adjuvant molecules represent a promising strategy to enhance tolerance induction. Until now, the development of allergy vaccines has been exclusively based on natural or modified allergen extracts, but, there is a growing interest in using recombinant allergens including native or hypoallergenic forms, mixture of allergens or allergen-derived peptides (Niederberger et al. 2004; Gafvelin et al. 2005; Purohit et al. 2008; Jutel et al. 2005; Muller et al. 1998; Himly et al. 2009; Pauli et al. 2008; Verhoef et al. 2005; Larche and Wraith 2005; Edlmayr et al. 2009). Thus, the development of relevant recombinant major allergens together with appropriate presentation systems suitable for mucosal application will help to develop more efficient and safe allergy vaccines in the future.

References

Allakhverdi Z, Fitzpatrick D, Boisvert A et al (2006) Expression of CD103 identifies human regulatory T-cell subsets. J Allergy Clin Immunol 118:1342–1349

Allam JP, Novak N, Fuchs C et al (2003) Characterization of dendritic cells from human oral mucosa: a new Langerhans' cell type with high constitutive FcεRI expression. J Allergy Clin Immunol 112:141–148

Allam JP, Peng WM, Appel T et al (2008a) Toll-like receptor 4 ligation enforces tolerogenic properties of oral mucosal Langerhans cells. J Allergy Clin Immunol 121:368–374 e1

Allam JP, Stojanovski G, Friedrichs N et al (2008b) Distribution of Langerhans cells and mast cells within the human oral mucosa: new application sites of allergens in sublingual immunotherapy? Allergy 63:720–727

Andri L, Falagiani P (2003) Symptomatic relief after grass nasal immunotherapy: lasting efficacy after 4–5 years. J Investig Allergol Clin Immunol 13:228–231

Andri L, Senna G (1995) Local nasal immunotherapy. Allergy 50:190

Andri L, Senna GE, Betteli C et al (1992) Local nasal immunotherapy in allergic rhinitis to Parietaria. A double-blind controlled study. Allergy 47:318–323

Andri L, Senna G, Betteli C et al (1993) Local nasal immunotherapy for Dermatophagoides-induced rhinitis: efficacy of a powder extract. J Allergy Clin Immunol 91:987–996

Andri L, Senna G, Betteli C et al (1996) Local nasal immunotherapy with extract in powder form is effective and safe in grass pollen rhinitis: a double-blind study. J Allergy Clin Immunol 97:34–41

Antunez C, Mayorga C, Corzo JL, Jurado A, Torres MJ (2008) Two year follow-up of immunological response in mite-allergic children treated with sublingual immunotherapy. Comparison with subcutaneous administration. Pediatr Allergy Immunol 19:210–218

Baena-Cagnani CE, Passalacqua G, Baena-Cagnani RC, Croce VH, Canonica WG (2005) Sublingual immunotherapy in pediatric patients: beyond clinical efficacy. Curr Opin Allergy Clin Immunol 5:173–177

Bagnasco M, Mariani G, Passalacqua G et al (1997) Absorption and distribution kinetics of the major Parietaria judaica allergen (Par j 1) administered by noninjectable routes in healthy human beings. J Allergy Clin Immunol 100:122–129

Bahceciler NN, Arikan C, Taylor A et al (2005) Impact of sublingual immunotherapy on specific antibody levels in asthmatic children allergic to house dust mites. Int Arch Allergy Immunol 136:287–294

Bellussi L, Bologna M, Di Stanislao C et al (2002) Simplified local nasal immunotherapy in mite dust allergic rhinitis. J Investig Allergol Clin Immunol 12:42–47

Benjaponpitak S, Oro A, Maguire P et al (1999) The kinetics of change in cytokine production by CD4 T cells during conventional allergen immunotherapy. J Allergy Clin Immunol 103:468–475

Bohle B, Breitwieser A, Zwolfer B et al (2004) A novel approach to specific allergy treatment: the recombinant fusion protein of a bacterial cell surface (S-layer) protein and the major birch pollen allergen Bet v 1 (rSbsC-Bet v 1) combines reduced allergenicity with immunomodulating capacity. J Immunol 172:6642–6648

Bohle B, Kinaciyan T, Gerstmayr M et al (2007) Sublingual immunotherapy induces IL-10-producing T regulatory cells, allergen-specific T-cell tolerance, and immune deviation. J Allergy Clin Immunol 120:707–713

Bonifaz LC, Bonnyay DP, Charalambous A et al (2004) In vivo targeting of antigens to maturing dendritic cells via the DEC-205 receptor improves T cell vaccination. J Exp Med 199: 815–824

Bousquet J, Lockey R, Malling HJ (1998) Allergen immunotherapy: therapeutic vaccines for allergic diseases. A WHO position paper. J Allergy Clin Immunol 102:558–562

Bousquet J, Scheinmann P, Guinnepain MT et al (1999) Sublingual-swallow immunotherapy (SLIT) in patients with asthma due to house-dust mites: a double-blind, placebo-controlled study. Allergy 54:249–260

Bousquet J, Van Cauwenberge P, Khaltaev N (2001) Allergic rhinitis and its impact on asthma. J Allergy Clin Immunol 108:S147–S334

Buchanan AD, Green TD, Jones SM et al (2007) Egg oral immunotherapy in nonanaphylactic children with egg allergy. J Allergy Clin Immunol 119:199–205

Burks AW, Laubach S, Jones SM (2008) Oral tolerance, food allergy, and immunotherapy: implications for future treatment. J Allergy Clin Immunol 121:1344–1350

Calamita Z, Saconato H, Pela AB, Atallah AN (2006) Efficacy of sublingual immunotherapy in asthma: systematic review of randomized-clinical trials using the Cochrane Collaboration method. Allergy 61:1162–1172

Canonica GW, Passalacqua G (2003) Noninjection routes for immunotherapy. J Allergy Clin Immunol 111:437–448 quiz 49

Chen ML, Yan BS, Bando Y, Kuchroo VK, Weiner HL (2008) Latency-associated peptide identifies a novel $CD4^{+}CD25^{+}$ regulatory T cell subset with TGFbeta-mediated function and enhanced suppression of experimental autoimmune encephalomyelitis. J Immunol 180:7327–7337

Ciprandi G, Fenoglio D, Cirillo I et al (2005) Induction of interleukin 10 by sublingual immunotherapy for house dust mites: a preliminary report. Ann Allergy Asthma Immunol 95:38–44

Clavel R, Bousquet J, Andre C (1998) Clinical efficacy of sublingual-swallow immunotherapy: a double-blind, placebo-controlled trial of a standardized five-grass-pollen extract in rhinitis. Allergy 53:493–498

Conti HR, Shen F, Nayyar N et al (2009) Th17 cells and IL-17 receptor signaling are essential for mucosal host defense against oral candidiasis. J Exp Med 206:299–311

Cosmi L, Santarlasci V, Angeli R et al (2006) Sublingual immunotherapy with Dermatophagoides monomeric allergoid down-regulates allergen-specific immunoglobulin E and increases both interferon-gamma- and interleukin 10-production. Clin Exp Allergy 36:261–272

Cuburu N, Kweon MN, Song JH et al (2007) Sublingual immunization induces broad-based systemic and mucosal immune responses in mice. Vaccine 25:8598–8610

D'Amato G, Lobefalo G, Liccardi G, Cazzola M (1995) A double-blind, placebo-controlled trial of local nasal immunotherapy in allergic rhinitis to Parietaria pollen. Clin Exp Allergy 25:141–148

Dahl R, Kapp A, Colombo G et al (2006) Efficacy and safety of sublingual immunotherapy with grass allergen tablets for seasonal allergic rhinoconjunctivitis. J Allergy Clin Immunol 118:434–440

Dahl R, Kapp A, Colombo G et al (2008) Sublingual grass allergen tablet immunotherapy provides sustained clinical benefit with progressive immunologic changes over 2 years. J Allergy Clin Immunol 121:512–518 e2

Daniel C, Repa A, Wild C et al (2006) Modulation of allergic immune responses by mucosal application of recombinant lactic acid bacteria producing the major birch pollen allergen Bet v 1. Allergy 61:812–819

Denning TL, Wang YC, Patel SR, Williams IR, Pulendran B (2007) Lamina propria macrophages and dendritic cells differentially induce regulatory and interleukin 17-producing T cell responses. Nat Immunol 8:1086–1094

Deuschl H, Johansson GO (1977) Hyposensitization of patients with allergic rhinitis by intranasal administration of chemically modified grass pollen allergen. A pilot study. Acta Allergol 32:248–262

Didier A, Melac M, Combebias A, Andre C (2006) Efficacy and safety of sublingual immunotherapy grass pollen tablets in grass pollen rhinoconjonctivitis. J Allergy Clin Immunol 117(Suppl LB5):721

Didier A, Melac M, Montagut A et al (2009) Agreement of efficacy assessments for five-grass pollen sublingual tablet immunotherapy. Allergy 64:166–171

Drachenberg KJ, Wheeler AW, Stuebner P, Horak F (2001) A well-tolerated grass pollen-specific allergy vaccine containing a novel adjuvant, monophosphoryl lipid A, reduces allergic symptoms after only four preseasonal injections. Allergy 56:498–505

Drachenberg KJ, Heinzkill M, Urban E, Woroniecki SR (2003) Efficacy and tolerability of short-term specific immunotherapy with pollen allergoids adjuvanted by monophosphoryl lipid A (MPL) for children and adolescents. Allergol Immunopathol (Madr) 31:270–277

Durham SR, Till SJ (1998) Immunologic changes associated with allergen immunotherapy. J Allergy Clin Immunol 102:157–164

Ebner C, Siemann U, Bohle B et al (1997) Immunological changes during specific immunotherapy of grass pollen allergy: reduced lymphoproliferative responses to allergen and shift from TH2 to TH1 in T-cell clones specific for Phl p 1, a major grass pollen allergen. Clin Exp Allergy 27:1007–1015

Edlmayr J, Niespodziana K, Linhart B et al (2009) A combination vaccine for allergy and rhinovirus infections based on rhinovirus-derived surface protein VP1 and a nonallergenic peptide of the major timothy grass pollen allergen Phl p 1. J Immunol 182:6298–6306

El Azami El Idrissi M, Ladant D, Leclerc C (2002) The adenylate cyclase of Bordetella pertussis: a vector to target antigen presenting cells. Toxicon 40:1661–1665

El Biaze M, Boniface S, Koscher V et al (2003) T cell activation, from atopy to asthma: more a paradox than a paradigm. Allergy 58:844–853

Faria AM, Weiner HL (2005) Oral tolerance. Immunol Rev 206:232–259

Faria AM, Weiner HL (2006a) Oral tolerance: therapeutic implications for autoimmune diseases. Clin Dev Immunol 13:143–157

Faria AM, Weiner HL (2006b) Oral tolerance and TGF-beta-producing cells. Inflamm Allergy Drug Targets 5:179–190

Fiocchi A, Pajno G, La Grutta S et al (2005) Safety of sublingual-swallow immunotherapy in children aged 3–7 years. Ann Allergy Asthma Immunol 95:254–258

Gafvelin G, Thunberg S, Kronqvist M et al (2005) Cytokine and antibody responses in birch-pollen-allergic patients treated with genetically modified derivatives of the major birch pollen allergen Bet v 1. Int Arch Allergy Immunol 138:59–66

Gardner LM, Thien FC, Douglass JA, Rolland JM, O'Hehir RE (2004) Induction of T 'regulatory' cells by standardized house dust mite immunotherapy: an increase in $CD4^+$ $CD25^+$ interleukin-10+ T cells expressing peripheral tissue trafficking markers. Clin Exp Allergy 34:1209–1219

Gehlhar K, Schlaak M, Becker W, Bufe A (1999) Monitoring allergen immunotherapy of pollen-allergic patients: the ratio of allergen-specific IgG4 to IgG1 correlates with clinical outcome. Clin Exp Allergy 29:497–506

Georgitis JW, Reisman RE, Clayton WF et al (1983) Local intranasal immunotherapy for grass-allergic rhinitis. J Allergy Clin Immunol 71:71–76

Giovane AL, Bardare M, Passalacqua G et al (1994) A three year double-blind placebo-controlled study with specific oral immunotherapy to Dermatophagoides: evidence of safety and efficacy in paediatric patients. Clin Exp Allergy 24:53–59

Goetsch L, Gonzalez A, Plotnicky-Gilquin H et al (2001) Targeting of nasal mucosa-associated antigen-presenting cells in vivo with an outer membrane protein A derived from *Klebsiella pneumoniae*. Infect Immun 69:6434–6444

Haicheur N, Benchetrit F, Amessou M et al (2003) The B subunit of Shiga toxin coupled to full-size antigenic protein elicits humoral and cell-mediated immune responses associated with a Th1-dominant polarization. Int Immunol 15:1161–1171

Hamid QA, Schotman E, Jacobson MR, Walker SM, Durham SR (1997) Increases in IL-12 messenger RNA+ cells accompany inhibition of allergen-induced late skin responses after successful grass pollen immunotherapy. J Allergy Clin Immunol 99:254–260

Hawiger D, Inaba K, Dorsett Y et al (2001) Dendritic cells induce peripheral T cell unresponsiveness under steady state conditions in vivo. J Exp Med 194:769–779

Himly M, Nony E, Chabre H et al (2009) Standardization of allergen products: 1. Detailed characterization of GMP-produced recombinant Bet v 1.0101 as biological reference preparation. Allergy 64(7):1038–1045

Hisbergues M, Magi M, Rigaux P et al (2007) In vivo and in vitro immunomodulation of Der p 1 allergen-specific response by Lactobacillus plantarum bacteria. Clin Exp Allergy 37:1286–1295

Horak F, Jaeger S, Worm M, Melac M, Didier A (2009) Implementation of pre-seasonal sublingual immunotherapy with a five-grass pollen tablet during optimal dosage assessment. Clin Exp Allergy 39:394–400

Huang FP, Platt N, Wykes M et al (2000) A discrete subpopulation of dendritic cells transports apoptotic intestinal epithelial cells to T cell areas of mesenteric lymph nodes. J Exp Med 191:435–444

Hufnagl K, Focke M, Gruber F et al (2008) Airway inflammation induced after allergic poly-sensitization can be prevented by mucosal but not by systemic administration of poly-peptides. Clin Exp Allergy 38:1192–1202

Ibanez MD, Kaiser F, Knecht R et al (2007) Safety of specific sublingual immunotherapy with SQ standardized grass allergen tablets in children. Pediatr Allergy Immunol 18:516–522

Iwasaki A, Kelsall BL (1999) Freshly isolated Peyer's patch, but not spleen, dendritic cells produce interleukin 10 and induce the differentiation of T helper type 2 cells. J Exp Med 190:229–239

Jeannin P, Renno T, Goetsch L et al (2000) OmpA targets dendritic cells, induces their maturation and delivers antigen into the MHC class I presentation pathway. Nat Immunol 1:502–509

Jonuleit H, Schmitt E, Schuler G, Knop J, Enk AH (2000) Induction of interleukin 10-producing, nonproliferating CD4(+) T cells with regulatory properties by repetitive stimulation with allogeneic immature human dendritic cells. J Exp Med 192:1213–1222

Jutel M, Akdis M, Budak F et al (2003) IL-10 and TGF-beta cooperate in the regulatory T cell response to mucosal allergens in normal immunity and specific immunotherapy. Eur J Immunol 33:1205–1214

Jutel M, Jaeger L, Suck R et al (2005) Allergen-specific immunotherapy with recombinant grass pollen allergens. J Allergy Clin Immunol 116:608–613

Khinchi MS, Poulsen LK, Carat F et al (2004) Clinical efficacy of sublingual and subcutaneous birch pollen allergen-specific immunotherapy: a randomized, placebo-controlled, double-blind, double-dummy study. Allergy 59:45–53

La Rosa M, Ranno C, Andre C et al (1999) Double-blind placebo-controlled evaluation of sublingual-swallow immunotherapy with standardized Parietaria judaica extract in children with allergic rhinoconjunctivitis. J Allergy Clin Immunol 104:425–432

Larche M (2000) Specific immunotherapy. Br Med Bull 56:1019–1036

Larche M, Wraith DC (2005) Peptide-based therapeutic vaccines for allergic and autoimmune diseases. Nat Med 11:S69–S76

Larenas-Linnemann D (2009) Sublingual immunotherapy in children: complete and updated review supporting evidence of effect. Curr Opin Allergy Clin Immunol 9:168–176

Lee SE, Koh YI, Kim MK et al (2008) Inhibition of airway allergic disease by co-administration of flagellin with allergen. J Clin Immunol 28:157–165

Leng X, Fu YX, Ye ST, Duan SQ (1990) A double-blind trial of oral immunotherapy for Artemisia pollen asthma with evaluation of bronchial response to the pollen allergen and serum-specific IgE antibody. Ann Allergy 64:27–31

Litwin A, Flanagan M, Entis G et al (1997) Oral immunotherapy with short ragweed extract in a novel encapsulated preparation: a double-blind study. J Allergy Clin Immunol 100:30–38

Liu YH, Tsai JJ (2005) Production of salivary immunoglobulin A and suppression of Dermatophagoides pteronyssinus-induced airway inflammation by local nasal immunotherapy. Int Arch Allergy Immunol 138:161–168

Liu L, Zhang M, Jenkins C, MacPherson GG (1998) Dendritic cell heterogeneity in vivo: two functionally different dendritic cell populations in rat intestinal lymph can be distinguished by CD4 expression. J Immunol 161:1146–1155
Lombardi V, Van Overtvelt L, Horiot S et al (2008) Toll-like receptor 2 agonist Pam3CSK4 enhances the induction of antigen-specific tolerance via the sublingual route. Clin Exp Allergy 38(11):1819–1829
Longo G, Barbi E, Berti I et al (2008) Specific oral tolerance induction in children with very severe cow's milk-induced reactions. J Allergy Clin Immunol 121:343–347
MacPherson G, Milling S, Yrlid U et al (2004) Uptake of antigens from the intestine by dendritic cells. Ann N Y Acad Sci 1029:75–82
Malling HJ, Montagut A, Melac M et al (2009) Efficacy and safety of five-grass pollen sublingual immunotherapy tablets in patients with different clinical profiles of allergic rhinoconjunctivitis. Clin Exp Allergy 39:387–393
Marcucci F, Sensi L, Frati F et al (2001) Sublingual tryptase and ECP in children treated with grass pollen sublingual immunotherapy (SLIT): safety and immunologic implications. Allergy 56:1091–1095
Marcucci F, Sensi L, Frati F et al (2003) Effects on inflammation parameters of a double-blind, placebo controlled 1 year course of SLIT in children monosensitized to mites. Allergy 58:657–662
Marcucci F, Sensi L, Incorvaia C et al (2007) Oral reactions to sublingual immunotherapy: a bioptic study. Allergy 62:1475–1477
Marogna M, Spadolini I, Massolo A, Canonica GW, Passalacqua G (2005) Clinical, functional, and immunologic effects of sublingual immunotherapy in birch pollinosis: a 3 year randomized controlled study. J Allergy Clin Immunol 115:1184–1188
Mascarell L, Van Overtvelt L, Moingeon P (2006) Novel ways for immune intervention in immunotherapy: mucosal allergy vaccines. Immunol Allergy Clin North Am 26:283–306 vii–viii
Mascarell L, Van Overtvelt L, Lombardi V et al (2007) A synthetic triacylated pseudo-dipeptide molecule promotes Th1/TReg immune responses and enhances tolerance induction via the sublingual route. Vaccine 26:108–118
Mascarell L, Lombardi V, Louise A et al (2008) Oral dendritic cells mediate antigen-specific tolerance by stimulating TH1 and regulatory $CD4^{+}$ T cells. J Allergy Clin Immunol 122:603–609 e5
Mascarell L, Lombardi V, Zimmer A et al (2009) Mapping of the lingual immune system reveals the presence of both regulatory and effector $CD4^{+}$ T cells. Clin Exp Allergy
Mavroleon G (1998) Restoration of cytokine imbalance by immunotherapy. Clin Exp Allergy 28:917–920
Medicines CoSo (1986) Desensitising vaccines: an allergist's view. Br Med J 293:1169–1170
Meglio P, Bartone E, Plantamura M, Arabito E (2004) Giampietro PG: A protocol for oral desensitization in children with IgE-mediated cow's milk allergy. Allergy 59:980–987
Meglio P, Giampietro PG, Gianni S, Galli E (2008) Oral desensitization in children with immunoglobulin E-mediated cow's milk allergy-follow-up at 4 year and 8 months. Pediatr Allergy Immunol 19:412–419
Meiler F, Zumkehr J, Klunker S et al (2008) In vivo switch to IL-10-secreting T regulatory cells in high dose allergen exposure. J Exp Med 205:2887–2898
Menges M, Rossner S, Voigtlander C et al (2002) Repetitive injections of dendritic cells matured with tumor necrosis factor alpha induce antigen-specific protection of mice from autoimmunity. J Exp Med 195:15–21
Michils A, Mairesse M, Ledent C et al (1998) Modified antigenic reactivity of anti-phospholipase A2 IgG antibodies in patients allergic to bee venom: conversion with immunotherapy and relation to subclass expression. J Allergy Clin Immunol 102:118–126
Moller C, Dreborg S, Lanner A, Bjorksten B (1986) Oral immunotherapy of children with rhinoconjunctivitis due to birch pollen allergy. A double blind study. Allergy 41:271–279

Moller C, Dreborg S, Ferdousi HA et al (2002) Pollen immunotherapy reduces the development of asthma in children with seasonal rhinoconjunctivitis (the PAT-study). J Allergy Clin Immunol 109:251–256

Mosbech H, Dreborg S, Madsen F et al (1987) High dose grass pollen tablets used for hyposensitization in hay fever patients. A one year double blind placebo-controlled study. Allergy 42:451–455

Mousavi T, Tajik N, Moradi M, Radjabzadeh MF (2008) CpG Immunotherapy in Chenopodium album sensitized mice: The comparison of IFN-gamma, IL-10 and IgE responses in intranasal and subcutaneous administrations. Clin Mol Allergy 6:10

Muller U, Akdis CA, Fricker M et al (1998) Successful immunotherapy with T-cell epitope peptides of bee venom phospholipase A2 induces specific T-cell anergy in patients allergic to bee venom. J Allergy Clin Immunol 101:747–754

Nakamura K, Kitani A, Strober W (2001) Cell contact-dependent immunosuppression by CD4(+)CD25(+) regulatory T cells is mediated by cell surface-bound transforming growth factor beta. J Exp Med 194:629–644

Nickelsen JA, Goldstein S, Mueller U et al (1981a) Local intranasal immunotherapy for ragweed allergic rhinitis. I. Clinical response. J Allergy Clin Immunol 68:33–40

Nickelsen JA, Goldstein S, Mueller U et al (1981b) Local intranasal immunotherapy for ragweed allergic rhinitis. II. Immunologic response. J Allergy Clin Immunol 68:41–45

Nickelsen JA, Georgitis JW, Mueller UR et al (1983) Local nasal immunotherapy for ragweed-allergic rhinitis. III. A two year of treatment. Clin Allergy 13:509–519

Niederberger V, Horak F, Vrtala S et al (2004) Vaccination with genetically engineered allergens prevents progression of allergic disease. Proc Natl Acad Sci U S A 101(Suppl 2):14677–14682

Novak N, Bieber T, Katoh N (2001) Engagement of Fc epsilon RI on human monocytes induces the production of IL-10 and prevents their differentiation in dendritic cells. J Immunol 167:797–804

Oida T, Zhang X, Goto M et al (2003) CD4+CD25- T cells that express latency-associated peptide on the surface suppress CD4+CD45RB high-induced colitis by a TGF-beta-dependent mechanism. J Immunol 170:2516–2522

Olaguibel JM, Alvarez Puebla MJ (2005) Efficacy of sublingual allergen vaccination for respiratory allergy in children. Conclusions from one meta-analysis. J Investig Allergol Clin Immunol 15:9–16

Pajno GB, Morabito L, Barberio G, Parmiani S (2000) Clinical and immunologic effects of long-term sublingual immunotherapy in asthmatic children sensitized to mites: a double-blind, placebo-controlled study. Allergy 55:842–849

Pajno GB, Peroni DG, Vita D et al (2003) Safety of sublingual immunotherapy in children with asthma. Paediatr Drugs 5:777–781

Passalacqua G, Albano M, Riccio AM, Scordamaglia A, Canonica GW (1997) Local nasal immunotherapy: experimental evidences and general considerations. Allergy 52:10–16

Passalacqua G, Albano M, Fregonese L et al (1998) Randomised controlled trial of local allergoid immunotherapy on allergic inflammation in mite-induced rhinoconjunctivitis. Lancet 351:629–632

Passalacqua G, Guerra L, Pasquali M, Lombardi C, Canonica GW (2004) Efficacy and safety of sublingual immunotherapy. Ann Allergy Asthma Immunol 93:3–12 quiz 12-3, 103

Passalacqua G, Altrinetti V, Mariani G et al (2005) Pharmacokinetics of radiolabelled Par j 1 administered intranasally to allergic and healthy subjects. Clin Exp Allergy 35:880–883

Patriarca G, Nucera E, Roncallo C et al (2003) Oral desensitizing treatment in food allergy: clinical and immunological results. Aliment Pharmacol Ther 17:459–465

Pauli G, Larsen TH, Rak S et al (2008) Efficacy of recombinant birch pollen vaccine for the treatment of birch-allergic rhinoconjunctivitis. J Allergy Clin Immunol 122:951–960

Penagos M, Compalati E, Tarantini F et al (2006) Efficacy of sublingual immunotherapy in the treatment of allergic rhinitis in pediatric patients 3–18 years of age: a meta-analysis of randomized, placebo-controlled, double-blind trials. Ann Allergy Asthma Immunol 97:141–148

Pichler CE, Pichler WJ (2001) Three years of specific immunotherapy with house-dust-mite extracts in patients with rhinitis and asthma: significant improvement of allergen-specific parameters and of nonspecific bronchial hyperreactivity. Allergy 56:301–306

Pierson-Mullany LK, Jackola D, Blumenthal M (2000) Rosenberg A: Altered allergen binding capacities of Amb a 1-specific IgE and IgG4 from ragweed-sensitive patients receiving immunotherapy. Ann Allergy Asthma Immunol 84:241–243

Powell RJ, Frew AJ, Corrigan CJ (2007) Durham SR: Effect of grass pollen immunotherapy with Alutard SQ on quality of life in seasonal allergic rhinoconjunctivitis. Allergy 62:1335–1338

Pugh CW, MacPherson GG, Steer HW (1983) Characterization of nonlymphoid cells derived from rat peripheral lymph. J Exp Med 157:1758–1779

Purohit A, Niederberger V, Kronqvist M et al (2008) Clinical effects of immunotherapy with genetically modified recombinant birch pollen Bet v 1 derivatives. Clin Exp Allergy 38:1514–1525

Radulovic S, Jacobson MR, Durham SR, Nouri-Aria KT (2008) Grass pollen immunotherapy induces Foxp3-expressing CD4+ CD25+ cells in the nasal mucosa. J Allergy Clin Immunol 121:1467–1472, 72 e1

Razafindratsita A, Saint-Lu N, Mascarell L et al (2007) Improvement of sublingual immunotherapy efficacy with a mucoadhesive allergen formulation. J Allergy Clin Immunol 120:278–285

Rebien W, Puttonen E, Maasch HJ, Stix E, Wahn U (1982) Clinical and immunological response to oral and subcutaneous immunotherapy with grass pollen extracts. A prospective study. Eur J Pediatr 138:341–344

Robinson DS, Larche M, Durham SR (2004) Tregs and allergic disease. J Clin Invest 114:1389–1397

Saint-Lu N, Tourdot S, Razafindratsita A et al (2009) Targeting the allergen to oral dendritic cells with mucoadhesive chitosan particles enhances tolerance induction. Allergy 64:1003–1013

Santeliz JV, Van Nest G, Traquina P, Larsen E, Wills-Karp M (2002) Amb a 1-linked CpG oligodeoxynucleotides reverse established airway hyperresponsiveness in a murine model of asthma. J Allergy Clin Immunol 109:455–462

Secrist H, Chelen CJ, Wen Y, Marshall JD, Umetsu DT (1993) Allergen immunotherapy decreases interleukin 4 production in CD4+ T cells from allergic individuals. J Exp Med 178:2123–2130

Simons FE, Shikishima Y, Van Nest G, Eiden JJ, HayGlass KT (2004) Selective immune redirection in humans with ragweed allergy by injecting Amb a 1 linked to immunostimulatory DNA. J Allergy Clin Immunol 113:1144–1151

Skripak JM, Nash SD, Rowley H et al (2008) A randomized, double-blind, placebo-controlled study of milk oral immunotherapy for cow's milk allergy. J Allergy Clin Immunol 122:1154–1160

Song JH, Nguyen HH, Cuburu N et al (2008) Sublingual vaccination with influenza virus protects mice against lethal viral infection. Proc Natl Acad Sci U S A 105:1644–1649

Staden U, Rolinck-Werninghaus C, Brewe F et al (2007) Specific oral tolerance induction in food allergy in children: efficacy and clinical patterns of reaction. Allergy 62:1261–1269

Steinman RM, Hawiger D, Liu K et al (2003) Dendritic cell function in vivo during the steady state: a role in peripheral tolerance. Ann N Y Acad Sci 987:15–25

Suffia I, Reckling SK, Salay G, Belkaid Y (2005) A role for CD103 in the retention of CD4+CD25+ Treg and control of Leishmania major infection. J Immunol 174:5444–5455

Sun CM, Hall JA, Blank RB et al (2007) Small intestine lamina propria dendritic cells promote de novo generation of Foxp3 T reg cells via retinoic acid. J Exp Med 204:1775–1785

Sun JB, Flach CF, Czerkinsky C, Holmgren J (2008) B lymphocytes promote expansion of regulatory T cells in oral tolerance: powerful induction by antigen coupled to cholera toxin B subunit. J Immunol 181:8278–8287

Taudorf E, Weeke B (1983) Orally administered grass pollen. Allergy 38:561–564

Taudorf E, Laursen LC, Lanner A et al (1987) Oral immunotherapy in birch pollen hay fever. J Allergy Clin Immunol 80:153–161

Taudorf E, Laursen L, Lanner A et al (1989) Specific IgE, IgG, and IgA antibody response to oral immunotherapy in birch pollinosis. J Allergy Clin Immunol 83:589–594

Taylor A, Verhagen J, Akdis CA, Akdis M (2004) T regulatory cells in allergy and health: a question of allergen specificity and balance. Int Arch Allergy Immunol 135:73–82

Tighe H, Takabayashi K, Schwartz D et al (2000) Conjugation of immunostimulatory DNA to the short ragweed allergen amb a 1 enhances its immunogenicity and reduces its allergenicity. J Allergy Clin Immunol 106:124–134

Tsai JJ, Liao EC, Tsai FH, Hsieh CC, Lee MF (2009) The effect of local nasal immunotherapy in allergic rhinitis: using strips of the allergen dermatophagoides pteronyssinus. J Asthma 46:165–170

Urbanek R, Burgelin KH, Kahle S, Kuhn W, Wahn U (1990) Oral immunotherapy with grass pollen in enterosoluble capsules. A prospective study of the clinical and immunological response. Eur J Pediatr 149:545–550

Van Overtvelt L, Lombardi V, Razafindratsita A et al (2008) IL-10-inducing adjuvants enhance sublingual immunotherapy efficacy in a murine asthma model. Int Arch Allergy Immunol 145:152–162

Verhoef A, Alexander C, Kay AB, Larche M (2005) T cell epitope immunotherapy induces a CD4+ T cell population with regulatory activity. PLoS Med 2:e78

Vourdas D, Syrigou E, Potamianou P et al (1998) Double-blind, placebo-controlled evaluation of sublingual immunotherapy with standardized olive pollen extract in pediatric patients with allergic rhinoconjunctivitis and mild asthma due to olive pollen sensitization. Allergy 53:662–672

Wachholz PA (2003) Durham SR: Induction of 'blocking' IgG antibodies during immunotherapy. Clin Exp Allergy 33:1171–1174

Wahn U, Tabar A, Kuna P et al (2009) Efficacy and safety of five-grass-pollen sublingual immunotherapy tablets in pediatric allergic rhinoconjunctivitis. J Allergy Clin Immunol 123:160–166 e3

Wilson DR, Torres LI, Durham SR (2003) Sublingual immunotherapy for allergic rhinitis. Cochrane Database Syst Rev CD002893

Wilson DR, Lima MT, Durham SR (2005) Sublingual immunotherapy for allergic rhinitis: systematic review and meta-analysis. Allergy 60:4–12

Winkler B, Hufnagl K, Spittler A et al (2006) The role of Foxp3+ T cells in long-term efficacy of prophylactic and therapeutic mucosal tolerance induction in mice. Allergy 61:173–180

T Cell Epitope-Based Allergy Vaccines

Mark Larché

Abstract Specific immunotherapy (SIT) with extracts containing intact allergen molecules is clinically efficacious, but associated with frequent adverse events related to the allergic sensitization of the patient. As a result, treatment is initiated in an incremental dose fashion which ultimately achieves a plateau (maintenance dose) that may be continued for several years. Reduction of allergic adverse events may allow safer and more rapid treatment Thus, many groups have developed and evaluated strategies to reduce allergenicity whilst maintaining immunogenicity, the latter being required to achieve specific modulation of the immune response. Peptide immunotherapy can be used to target T and/or B cells in an antigen-specific manner. To date, only approaches that target T cells have been clinically evaluated. Short, synthetic peptides representing immunodominant T cell epitopes of major allergens are able to modulate allergen-specific T cell responses in the absence of IgE cross linking and activation of effector cells. Here we review clinical and mechanistic studies associated with peptide immunotherapy targeting allergy to cats or to bee venom.

Contents

M. Larché (✉)
Department of Medicine, Firestone Institute for Respiratory Health,
McMaster University, HSC 4H20, 1200 Main Street West,
Hamilton ON L8N 3Z5, Canada
e-mail: larche@mcmaster.ca

Current Topics in Microbiology and Immunology (2011) 352: 107–119
DOI: 10.1007/82_2011_131

Published Online: 13 May 2011

1 Introduction

Specific allergen immunotherapy as a clinical intervention is approaching its centenary year. Since the inception of controlled clinical trials of this therapeutic modality in the 1950s it has been widely demonstrated to be clinically effective and to have a duration of action that substantially exceeds the treatment period (Durham et al. 1999). The latter is indicative of the induction of functional immunological tolerance, although the precise mechanisms underlying such a phenomenon remain incompletely understood. Despite lasting clinical efficacy, current clinical practice with whole allergen extracts requires an extended period of treatment, the generally accepted optimum period being 3 years. The lengthy treatment period is caused, at least in part, by dose limitations related to the frequent occurrence of predominantly IgE-mediated adverse events. Adverse events are manifested as allergic reactions to the treatment and range from mild local reactions to severe systemic reactions including anaphylactic shock. A number of strategies aimed at reducing the allergenicity of treatment preparations whilst maintaining immunogenicity, has been described. Physical modification of allergen molecules offers the prospect of reducing or eliminating IgE reactivity and thus, allergenicity. Such approaches have taken many forms including chemical modification, conjugation with synthetic bacterial DNA motifs, point mutations in native allergen gene sequences, and the use of allergen multimers, fragments, and peptides of various lengths. The use of soluble synthetic peptides for the treatment of allergic disease allows the delivery of T cell epitopes of the allergen in a tolerogenic form, whilst avoiding IgE-mediated allergic reactions. Synthetic peptides have been evaluated in both experimental animal models and in human clinical studies. Synthetic peptides are defined chemical entities and can be produced and standardized to levels impossible to achieve with allergen extracts. Furthermore, they are inexpensive to produce, easy to purify and are stable in lyophilized form.

Early indications that peptides may be used to modulate immune responses toward tolerant phenotypes came from in vitro studies investigating the effects of high-dose peptide presentation between T cells. Pure populations of $CD4^+$ helper T cell clones were pre-treated with supraoptimal concentrations of specific peptide and subsequently shown to be refractory to antigen stimulation (Lamb et al. 1983). As antigen presenting cells were not present in the cultures, presentation of peptide to T cell receptors likely occurred through binding to MHC class II molecules on T cells and recognition of antigen in a "non-professional" context. Subsequent studies have confirmed the ability of non-professional antigen presenting cells to induce T cell tolerance (Bal et al. 1990).

Experimental in vivo studies of peptide-induced tolerance have been reported in a number of disease areas including allergy, autoimmunity, and transplantation. Initial experiments demonstrated that it was possible to induce systemic tolerance to peptides administered in incomplete Freund's adjuvant during the neonatal period (Gammon et al. 1986; Clayton et al. 1989). Several studies have focused on prevention and treatment of experimental autoimmune encephalomyelitis (EAE), a model of multiple sclerosis (MS) (Critchfield et al. 1994) (Gaur et al. 1992; Metzler and Wraith 1993). Recently in a T cell receptor transgenic model of EAE, MBP peptides were administered via the intranasal route leading to protection from disease, which required deletion of effector T cells and the presence of IL-10 (Burkhart et al. 1999; Anderton et al. 1998). Peptide therapy has also been shown to be effective in murine models of experimental arthritis (Ku et al. 1993; Staines et al. 1996; Prakken et al. 1997), and in models of type I diabetes (Daniel and Wegmann 1996; Bockova et al. 1997; Tian et al. 1996).

A limited number of in vivo studies of peptide therapy have been performed in models of allergic disease. Mice primed with the major house dust mite allergen Der p 2 were treated with peptides containing immunodominant T cell epitopes from Der p 2. T cell and B cell (antibody) responses to the protein were down-regulated (Hoyne et al. 1993). The dominant T cell epitope of the birch pollen allergen Bet v 1 was administered prophylactically and therapeutically to CBA/J mice and inhibited T cell responses without a detectable effect on antibody production (Bauer et al. 1997). Prophylactic treatment of venom sensitized mice with peptides from the bee venom allergen Api m4, or the hornet venom allergen Dol m 5, reduced T and B cell responses to allergen challenge (King et al. 1998). In another study of insect venom allergy, mice sensitized to Api m 1 (phospholipase A_2; PLA_2) were treated with a mixture of three polypeptides spanning the entire molecule. Mice were protected from anaphylaxis. A significant reduction in specific IgE was observed together with an increase in allergen-specific IgG2a and a reduced Th2:Th1 ratio (von Garnier et al. 2000). Mice sensitized to the major cat allergen Fel d 1 were treated with two allergen-derived polypeptides that encompassed much of the sequence of Fel d 1 chain 1. Treatment resulted in decreased production of IL-2 and allergen-specific IgG, but no Th2-specific outcomes were reported (Briner et al. 1993). Most recently, Campbell and colleagues sensitized mice devoid of murine MHC class II and transgenic for the human MHC molecule HLA-DRB1*0101, with recombinant Fel d 1 and subsequently treated them with a single ultra-low dose (1 μg) of a Fel d 1 peptide previously shown to bind to HLA-DRB1*0101. Treatment ameliorated allergic airways disease and suppressed the systemic Th2 response to allergen. Tolerance induced by this single T cell epitope was found to cross over to other T cell epitopes of Fel d 1, indicative of the induction of linked epitope suppression. Tolerance in this model was shown to be IL-10 dependent (Campbell et al. 2009).

Little is known about the most effective dose for induction of tolerance through peptide therapy. In mice, tolerogenic peptide doses range from a few microgrammes (Chai et al. 2004) to milligrammes (Karin et al. 1994). By delivering T cell epitopes directly to dendritic cells in vivo, it has recently been shown that doses of little as

500 pg can induce tolerance in a murine model (Kretschmer et al. 2005). Fundamental differences may exist in the mechanisms of low and high-dose tolerance. High-dose protocols have been associated with clonal deletion and, to a lesser extent, anergy of antigen-specific cells (Critchfield et al. 1994; Karin et al. 1994; Kearney et al. 1994). Fewer studies of low dose tolerance have been performed, but both high and low dose models appear to be characterized by the induction of T cells with regulatory activity (Wraith et al. 2003, 2004; Apostolou and Von Boehmer 2004).

2 Clinical Studies

To date, translation of peptide immunotherapy into the clinical setting has focused on the treatment of cat allergy and bee venom allergy. The earliest studies employed two polypeptides from the major cat allergen Fel d 1, these peptides having previously been evaluated in a murine model of cat allergy described above. In a study by Norman and colleagues, an equimolar mixture of the peptides (27 amino acids each in length; IPC-1/IPC-2) or placebo, was given in four subcutaneous injections, over a period of 2 weeks, to 95 cat-allergic subjects (all with allergic rhinitis to cats and some with asthma) in three dose groups (7.5, 75 and 750 μg per injection) (Norman et al. 1996). Statistically significant, albeit modest, improvements in lung and nasal symptom scores were observed, but only in the high-dose group. A large placebo effect was observed in common with many allergen immunotherapy trials. Treatment was associated with a significant incidence of adverse events, which occurred a few minutes to several hours after peptide injection. Most frequently, subjects with a history of asthma reported chest tightness and wheezing several hours after peptide administration. This phenomenon was later investigated and shown to be attributable to isolated late asthmatic reactions following MHC-restricted activation of allergen (peptide)-specific T cells in the airways (Haselden et al. 1999). Mechanistic in vitro studies associated with the Norman study demonstrated reduced IL-4 production in peptide-specific T cell lines following therapy suggesting a decrease in allergen-specific Th2 responses (Marcotte et al. 1998).

Pène and colleagues evaluated the same peptides in an inhaled allergen challenge study. A reduction in allergen PD_{20} (provocative dose of inhaled allergen resulting in a 20% reduction in forced expiratory volume in one second; FEV_1) was seen in both high and medium (individual doses of 75 μg up to a total dose of 450 μg–medium dose and 4,500 μg–high dose) dose groups when compared to baseline, but not placebo (Pene et al. 1998). In mechanistic studies peripheral blood mononuclear cells were stimulated with cat allergen in vitro, before and after treatment, a reduction in IL-4 production was reported (in the high dose group), in agreement with earlier findings.

In contrast to these studies that reported some clinical benefit from therapy, a third trial found no clinical effect. In a double-blind, parallel group study, Simons and colleagues gave weekly (total of four) subcutaneous injections, of 250 μg of the peptide mixture or placebo, to 42 subjects with cat-allergic rhinitis and/or asthma

(Simons et al. 1996). Treatment was associated with late onset symptoms of rhinitis, asthma, and pruritis. No changes in early and late-phase skin responses to intradermal allergen challenge were observed. In associated mechanistic studies, PBMC cytokine secretion was not different between peptide-treated and placebo-treated subjects.

In the last reported study with IPC-1/IPC-2, 133 cat-allergic subjects were treated in a multi-center study design. Each subject received eight subcutaneous injections of 750 μg. The only positive clinical effect observed was a significant improvement in pulmonary function, which was seen only in individuals with reduced baseline FEV_1 (Maguire et al. 1999). Furthermore, improvements in pulmonary function were evident at only a single time point (3 weeks) after therapy. Frequent adverse events were reported during treatment, including some requiring epinephrine. In common with other studies using these peptides, late onset adverse reactions (isolated late asthmatic reactions) diminished with successive doses of peptide indicating that immunological tolerance was being induced to the peptides. The reduction in magnitude and frequency of adverse events through induction of peptide-specific tolerance was presumably related to the clinical benefits reported in this series of studies.

More recently, a series of clinical studies have been performed using mixtures of shorter peptides from Fel d 1 (Oldfield et al. 2001, 2002; Alexander et al. 2005; Smith et al. 2004; Verhoef et al. 2005). Cat-allergic asthmatic volunteers were challenged intradermally with whole cat dander allergen extract, before and after a single injection of 5 μg of each of twelve peptides in saline. The peptides encompassed approximately 80% of the Fel d 1 molecule and contained most of the major T cell epitopes (unpublished observations). Intradermal peptide injection significantly reduced the magnitude of the cutaneous late-phase reaction to allergen challenge given approximately 2–4 weeks after baseline measurements. In vitro mechanistic studies with PBMC demonstrated reduced allergen-specific proliferation and a reduction in both Th1 and Th2 cytokines (Oldfield et al. 2001).

The same mixture of 12 peptides was then evaluated in a double-blind, placebo-controlled clinical trial (Oldfield et al. 2002). Twenty four cat-allergic asthmatic subjects with moderate to severe asthma (PC20 as low as 0.1 mg/ml histamine) were treated with 4–5 injections of increasing dose (lowest dose 5 μg; highest dose 50 μg). Quality of life was evaluated by questionnaire (Global evaluation to cat exposure visual analogue scale). The primary outcome measure of the study was the size of the late-phase cutaneous reaction to intradermal challenge with allergen. Secondary outcome measures included the early-phase cutaneous reaction to allergen challenge, the allergen PD_{20} and the histamine PC_{20}. Baseline measurements were compared to two post-treatment follow-up evaluations; 4–8 weeks after therapy and 3–9 months after therapy. Subjects received a total of 90 μg of each of 12 peptides in divided incremental doses administered at 3–4 day intervals. A statistically significant reduction in the magnitude of both early (second follow-up only) and late-phase cutaneous reactions (both follow-up assessments) to intradermal challenge with allergen when compared to placebo was recorded. In mechanistic studies, reduced proliferative responses and reduced Th1 and Th2 cytokine production following culture with allergen were observed. The reductions in pro-inflammatory cytokines were associated with an increase in production of IL-10. A recent publication (Campbell et al. 2009) also reported responses to individual peptides measured in PBMC samples from this study. The results showed that in addition to modulating the immune response to the vaccine peptides themselves, peptide therapy also modulated the immune response to non-injected peptides from the same allergen, indicative of intramolecular tolerance (also known as "linked epitope suppression"). Subjects treated with peptides felt significantly better able to tolerate exposure to cats after therapy although this improvement was not statistically significant when compared to the placebo group. No significant improvements were observed in PD_{20} or PC_{20}, however, the study was not powered to detect such changes. No immediate adverse events were reported in this study, but isolated late asthmatic reactions were expected (based on the dose of peptides employed) and recorded. Retrospective analysis of the incidence of these reactions and the induction of tolerance/improvement in outcomes, demonstrated that the induction of an isolated late asthmatic reaction was not required for the induction of tolerance.

In a related open-label study using a similar peptide preparation delivered at 2 week intervals and using a lower dosing regimen, a significant reduction in airway hyperreactivity (measured by PC_{20}) was observed (Alexander et al. 2005). Five incremental intradermal injections were given (0.1, 1.0, 5, 10, and 25 μg). A reduction in the cutaneous late-phase reaction to allergen challenge was also observed in common with other related studies. Immunohistochemistry of skin biopsy tissue obtained after allergen challenge revealed a significant increase in the number of $CD25^+$ cells and the number of $CD4^+$/IFN-γ^+ cells after peptide treatment, suggesting that recruitment of Th1 cells (and perhaps regulatory T cells) to the skin may be an important mechanism. No increase in IL-10^+ cells was observed in the skin but expression of TGFβ mRNA appeared to be increased but the cellular source of this cytokine could not be determined.

A related study aimed to investigate the effect of peptide immunotherapy on peripheral blood $CD4^+$ responses and $CD4^+CD25^+$ suppression of allergen-stimulated cultures in a double-blind, placebo-controlled trial (Smith et al. 2004). Proliferative responses and IL-13 production from PBMC cultured with allergen in vitro were significantly reduced following peptide therapy as in previous studies. The functional regulatory activity of $CD4^+CD25^+$ cells was assessed by mixing with autologous $CD4^+CD25^-$ cells. Peptide immunotherapy did not alter the suppressive activity of $CD4^+CD25^+$ cells in this study suggesting that naturally occurring regulatory T cells may not play a significant role in the immunological changes associated with peptide immunotherapy. Observations that may support this conclusion were made in a recent murine study which showed no increase in Fox p 3 + T cells in the lungs of mice after successful peptide therapy (Campbell et al. 2009).

A potential role of antigen-specific inducible regulatory T cells was addressed in a subsequent study by mixing $CD4^+$ T cells (containing the putative regulatory cells) with $CD4^-$ cells (Verhoef et al. 2005). Each population was labeled with a different fluorescent dye ($CD4^+$ were labeled red with PKH-26 and $CD4^-$ were labeled green with the cell cycle-tracking dye CFSE). In an autologous culture system, $CD4^+$ cells from before and after peptide therapy were mixed with $CD4^-$ cells from before and after therapy, in all possible combinations. The results showed that antigen-specific proliferative responses of memory T cells were reduced following peptide immunotherapy compared to baseline samples and that $CD4^+$ cells isolated after treatment could suppress the proliferative response of baseline $CD4^-$ cells. These data suggest that peptide immunotherapy can induce a population of $CD4^+$ T cells with suppressive/regulatory activity.

3 Insect Venom Allergy

Subcutaneous whole allergen immunotherapy for insect venom allergy is highly effective although it requires a protracted treatment period. Systemic adverse events are common during treatment, encouraging the development of therapies with reduced allergenicity, such as the peptide approach. Five bee venom allergic subjects received incremental doses of three immunodominant peptides (an equimolar mixture) at weekly (Muller et al. 1998). Ten control subjects were treated with conventional bee venom immunotherapy to compare clinical outcomes and mechanisms. The cumulative peptide dose was 397.1 μg. One week after the last peptide injection, subjects were challenged subcutaneously with 10 μg of whole Api m 1. All five subjects tolerated the challenge without systemic allergic symptoms. One week later a wild bee sting challenge was performed. Three out of five tolerated this challenge without reaction, the remaining two subjects developed mild systemic allergic reactions. However, due to the variable nature of the allergic response to bee stings, it is likely that as many as half of these individuals would not have had a severe reaction to the sting challenge regardless of treatment. No change was observed in levels of allergen-specific serum IgE or IgG_4 during the course of peptide therapy. Interestingly, following subcutaneous challenge with the whole allergen 1 week after the last peptide injection, concentrations of both isotypes increased sharply, particularly IgG_4 and a month later serum levels of specific IgG_4 were higher than IgE.

Immunodominant T cell epitopes of Api m 1 and their MHC restriction elements were determined by Texier and colleagues, by direct binding of peptides to purified MHC class II molecules (Texier et al. 2000). Four peptides were identified, three of which were similar to those used previously for therapy by Müller and colleagues. Following a similar treatment regimen to Müller, Tarzi and colleagues performed a controlled, open-label, single-blind study of peptide therapy in subjects with mild bee venom allergy (Tarzi et al. 2005). The peptides were well tolerated and no adverse events were observed during treatment. In mechanistic studies, PBMC responses to purified allergen and whole bee venom were significantly reduced. Proliferative responses to treatment peptides were also reduced. Th2 cytokine production following culture with allergen was reduced, but IL-10 production was significantly increased, confirming earlier findings in subjects treated with cat peptides. Late-phase cutaneous reactions to both whole bee venom and Api m 1 were significantly reduced following allergen challenge. Allergen-specific IgG, IgG_4 and IgE levels were measured using serum samples were collected before, during, and after treatment. A statistically significant, but transient, increase in allergen-specific IgG and IgG_4 during and after treatment was found. The functional significance of such an increase, which was considerably smaller in absolute terms than the response seen in whole allergen therapy, remains to be determined.

Using much larger peptides (long synthetic peptides; LSP) that encompassed the entire Api m 1 molecule, Fellrath and colleagues treated bee venom allergic subjects with a RUSH desensitization protocol (Fellrath et al. 2003). Patients received approximately 250 μg in incremental doses at 30 min intervals starting with 0.1 μg. Maintenance injections of 100 μg, or in some cases 300 μg, were given on days 4, 7, 14, 42 and 70. In the active treatment group a transient increase in T cell proliferation to the peptides was observed, together with an increase in IFNγ and IL-10 levels, but not Th2 cytokines. Allergen-specific IgG_4 but not IgE levels increased throughout the study period, similar to whole allergen therapy. Peptide-specific IgE was induced in some patients during the study. No significant change in skin sensitivity to intradermal allergen challenge was observed. Peptide therapy was generally well tolerated, however, local and disseminated erythema with hand (palm) pruritis was observed in two subjects.

4 Mechanisms of Peptide-Induced Tolerance

Peptide-induced tolerance following intradermal (systemic route) injection, is not replicated when peptides are administered via inhalation, despite the fact that both routes are equivalent in their ability to induce isolated late asthmatic reactions (Ali et al. 2004). Thus, T cell tolerance is likely to arise through systemic presentation of peptides (which in our own studies are delivered in saline, without adjuvant and at very low doses) to naïve T cells by non-professional APC (such as endothelial cells, epithelial cells etc.) and "steady-state" (quiescent) dendritic cells. All of these cell types are known to induce tolerogenic T cell responses (Steinman et al. 2003). Since the peptides are probably encountered in a non-inflammatory environment, the T cells probably make a "tolerant" response that leads to the expansion of existing allergen-specific regulatory T cells and de novo generation of more of these cells from the naïve T cell pool. When peptides are administered by intradermal injection, a significant amount of the injected dose is likely to pass rapidly into the systemic circulation through the capillary bed. Once in the circulation, peptides rapidly reach all tissues and bind to MHC class II molecules of the appropriate specificity. Relatively low plasma dose and high solubility may render peptides "tolerogenic". Recent studies have suggested that cross-linking of IgE on the surface of antigen presenting cells (for example, by allergen) results in the activation of these cells and the release of cytokines which may have a pro-inflammatory outcome (Novak et al. 2001). In contrast, the small size of peptides does not allow them to crosslink adjacent IgE molecules and it follows, therefore, that peptides will elicit less inflammation than whole allergen. Thus, peptides may bind to MHC class II molecules on the cell surface without activating the cell. Previous studies have demonstrated the presence of a significant percentage of "empty" MHC class II molecules on the surface of immature and "steady state" dendritic cells (Santambrogio et al. 1999a). Empty MHC molecules are also associated with active HLA-DM, a chaperone and peptide editing protein, that loads exogenous peptides into empty MHC class II binding grooves (Santambrogio et al. 1999b). As a result, when peptide-loaded dendritic cells recycle through lymphoid tissue, they will present peptides to T cells whilst in a quiescent state resulting in a tolerogenic encounter.

5 Future Peptide Vaccine Design

In those allergens in which extensive T cell epitope mapping studies have been performed, it is clear that most allergens contain large numbers of T cell epitopes distributed throughout the molecule. Issues of solubility and formulation of a mixture of peptides for immunotherapy mean that peptide vaccines are unlikely to be able to accommodate all T cell epitopes in an allergen. Thus, critical choices must be made regarding which epitopes are the most important. The recent description of linked epitope suppression following peptide therapy in both human and murine systems provides an immunological basis for how a small number of selected T cell epitopes might confer tolerance to all epitopes in an allergen molecule (Campbell et al. 2009). In some cases lack of solubility of linear synthetic peptides precludes their presence in a vaccine, despite the fact that these sequences do exist as processed T cell epitopes in vivo. Ideally, peptides must have the ability to bind to diverse HLA types representing a broad cross section of the population. They must not selectively induce Th2 cytokines that may enhance Th2 responses in vivo. If the mechanisms underlying conventional immunotherapy are similar to that of peptide vaccination then induction of IFN-γ and IL-10 (and perhaps TGFβ) is desirable. In addition, peptide should not induce IgE antibody production but promote the generation of inhibitory IgG antibodies. These ideals may underlie the protective effect of high-dose natural exposure to cat allergens as reported by Woodfolk and colleagues (Carneiro et al. 2004). Cat-allergic subjects, whilst having high allergen-specific IgE levels, also produce IgG4 which appeared to protect from disease. This was described as a "modified Th2 response". Analysis of particular peptides from Fel d1 suggested the preferential induction of IL-10 (Reefer et al. 2004). Such peptides should be included in future clinical trials of cat peptide vaccination to enhance vaccine efficiency.

6 Summary

Several strategies to reduce the allergenicity of therapeutic preparations for the treatment of allergic diseases are under development. Short, synthetic peptides containing T cell epitopes of clinically important major allergens show markedly reduced ability to crosslink allergen-specific IgE. In a number of clinical studies, peptide treatment has been shown to modify surrogate markers of allergen exposure such as; cutaneous responses to allergen challenge, bronchial hyperreactivity (some studies), symptoms scores following nasal allergen challenge, quality of life, and the ability to tolerate natural allergen exposure. Mechanistic studies indicate that peptide therapy induces both immune deviation (Th2–Th1 response) and regulatory T cells capable of suppressing allergen-specific immune responses. Limited data is available on the effects of peptide therapy on humoral immune responses. There appears to substantially less allergen-specific IgG induced during peptide therapy (compared to conventional allergen extract immunotherapy). Treatment with bee venom peptides appears to induce allergen-specific IgG4, but this may be induced by exposure to whole allergen after treatment (in the context of IL-10-rich T cell help) rather than by direct exposure to treatment peptides. The reduced size of peptides and relative lack of conformational determinants are associated with reduced basophil activation and histamine release in vitro. Intradermal delivery of short peptides has demonstrated a substantial reduction in allergenicity compared to comparable molar doses of whole allergen. It is expected that this reduced allergenicity will translate into a reduced risk of IgE-mediated adverse events such as anaphylaxis. It remains to be seen whether the clinical response to peptide immunotherapy will be of equivalent efficacy to conventional treatment. Further peptide therapy studies and comparisons with existing therapy are anticipated.

Acknowledgments The author is funded by the Canada Research Chairs program, a McMaster University/GlaxoSmithKline Chair in Lung Immunology at St. Joseph's Healthcare, the Canadian Institutes for Health Research, AllerGen Network of Centres of Excellence and the Canadian Foundation for Innovation.

References

Alexander C, Ying S, Kay B, Larche M (2005) Fel d 1-derived T cell peptide therapy induces recruitment of CD4CD25; CD4 interferon-gamma T helper type 1 cells to sites of allergen-induced late-phase skin reactions in cat-allergic subjects. Clin Exp Allergy 35(1):52–58

Ali FR, Oldfield WL, Higashi N, Larche M, Kay AB (2004) Late asthmatic reactions induced by inhalation of allergen-derived T cell peptides. Am J Respir Crit Care Med 169(1):20–26

Anderton SM, Burkhart C, Liu GY, Metzler B, Wraith DC (1998) Antigen-specific tolerance induction and the immunotherapy of experimental autoimmune disease. Novartis Found Symp 215:120–131

Apostolou I, Von Boehmer H (2004) In vivo instruction of suppressor commitment in naive T cells. J Exp Med 199(10):1401–1408

Bal V, McIndoe A, Denton G, Hudson D, Lombardi G, Lamb J et al (1990) Antigen presentation by keratinocytes induces tolerance in human T cells. Eur J Immunol 20(9):1893–1897

Bauer L, Bohle B, Jahn-Schmid B, Wiedermann U, Daser A, Renz H et al (1997) Modulation of the allergic immune response in BALB/c mice by subcutaneous injection of high doses of the dominant T cell epitope from the major birch pollen allergen Bet v 1. Clin Exp Immunol 107(3):536–541

Bockova J, Elias D, Cohen IR (1997) Treatment of NOD diabetes with a novel peptide of the hsp60 molecule induces Th2-type antibodies. J Autoimmun 10(4):323–329

Briner TJ, Kuo MC, Keating KM, Rogers BL, Greenstein JL (1993) Peripheral T-cell tolerance induced in naive and primed mice by subcutaneous injection of peptides from the major cat allergen Fel d I. Proc Natl Acad Sci USA 90(16):7608–7612

Burkhart C, Liu GY, Anderton SM, Metzler B, Wraith DC (1999) Peptide-induced T cell regulation of experimental autoimmune encephalomyelitis: a role for IL-10. Int Immunol 11(10):1625–1634

Campbell JD, Buckland KF, McMillan SJ, Kearley J, Oldfield WL, Stern LJ et al (2009) Peptide immunotherapy in allergic asthma generates IL-10-dependent immunological tolerance associated with linked epitope suppression. J Exp Med 206(7):1535–1547

Carneiro R, Reefer A, Wilson B, Hammer J, Platts-Mills T, Custis N et al (2004) T cell epitope-specific defects in the immune response to cat allergen in patients with atopic dermatitis. J Invest Dermatol 122(4):927–936

Chai JG, James E, Dewchand H, Simpson E, Scott D (2004) Transplantation tolerance induced by intranasal administration of HY peptides. Blood 103(10):3951–3959

Clayton JP, Gammon GM, Ando DG, Kono DH, Hood L, Sercarz EE (1989) Peptide-specific prevention of experimental allergic encephalomyelitis. Neonatal tolerance induced to the dominant T cell determinant of myelin basic protein J Exp Med 169(5):1681–1691

Critchfield JM, Racke MK, Zuniga-Pflucker JC, Cannella B, Raine CS, Goverman J et al (1994) T cell deletion in high antigen dose therapy of autoimmune encephalomyelitis. Science 263(5150):1139–1143

Daniel D, Wegmann DR (1996) Protection of nonobese diabetic mice from diabetes by intranasal or subcutaneous administration of insulin peptide B-(9-23). Proc Natl Acad Sci USA 93(2):956–960

Durham SR, Walker SM, Varga EM, Jacobson MR, O'Brien F, Noble W et al (1999) Long-term clinical efficacy of grass-pollen immunotherapy. N Engl J Med 341(7):468–475

Fellrath JM, Kettner A, Dufour N, Frigerio C, Schneeberger D, Leimgruber A et al (2003) Allergen-specific T-cell tolerance induction with allergen-derived long synthetic peptides: results of a phase I trial. J Allergy Clin Immunol 111(4):854–861

Gammon G, Dunn K, Shastri N, Oki A, Wilbur S, Sercarz EE (1986) Neonatal T-cell tolerance to minimal immunogenic peptides is caused by clonal inactivation. Nature 319(6052):413–415

Gaur A, Wiers B, Liu A, Rothbard J, Fathman CG (1992) Amelioration of autoimmune encephalomyelitis by myelin basic protein synthetic peptide-induced anergy. Science 258(5087):1491–1494

Haselden BM, Kay AB, Larche M (1999) Immunoglobulin E-independent major histocompatibility complex-restricted T cell peptide epitope-induced late asthmatic reactions. J Exp Med 189(12):1885–1894

Hoyne GF, O'Hehir RE, Wraith DC, Thomas WR, Lamb JR (1993) Inhibition of T cell and antibody responses to house dust mite allergen by inhalation of the dominant T cell epitope in naive and sensitized mice. J Exp Med 178(5):1783–1788

Karin N, Mitchell DJ, Brocke S, Ling N, Steinman L (1994) Reversal of experimental autoimmune encephalomyelitis by a soluble peptide variant of a myelin basic protein epitope: T cell receptor antagonism and reduction of interferon gamma and tumor necrosis factor alpha production. J Exp Med 180(6):2227–2237

Kearney ER, Pape KA, Loh DY, Jenkins MK (1994) Visualization of peptide-specific T cell immunity and peripheral tolerance induction in vivo. Immunity 1(4):327–339

King TP, Lu G, Agosto H (1998) Antibody responses to bee melittin (Api m 4) and hornet antigen 5 (Dol m 5) in mice treated with the dominant T-cell epitope peptides. J Allergy Clin Immunol 101(3):397–403

Kretschmer K, Apostolou I, Hawiger D, Khazaie K, Nussenzweig MC, Von Boehmer H (2005) Inducing and expanding regulatory T cell populations by foreign antigen. Nat Immunol 6:152–162

Ku G, Kronenberg M, Peacock DJ, Tempst P, Banquerigo ML, Braun BS et al (1993) Prevention of experimental autoimmune arthritis with a peptide fragment of type II collagen. Eur J Immunol 23(3):591–599

Lamb JR, Skidmore BJ, Green N, Chiller JM, Feldmann M (1983) Induction of tolerance in influenza virus-immune T lymphocyte clones with synthetic peptides of influenza hemagglutinin. J Exp Med 157(5):1434–1447

Maguire P, Nicodemus C, Robinson D, Aaronson D, Umetsu DT (1999) The safety and efficacy of ALLERVAX CAT in cat allergic patients. Clin Immunol 93(3):222–231

Marcotte GV, Braun CM, Norman PS, Nicodemus CF, Kagey-Sobotka A, Lichtenstein LM et al (1998) Effects of peptide therapy on ex vivo T-cell responses. J Allergy Clin Immunol 101(4 Pt 1):506–513

Metzler B, Wraith DC (1993) Inhibition of experimental autoimmune encephalomyelitis by inhalation but not oral administration of the encephalitogenic peptide: influence of MHC binding affinity. Int Immunol 5(9):1159–1165

Muller U, Akdis CA, Fricker M, Akdis M, Blesken T, Bettens F et al (1998) Successful immunotherapy with T-cell epitope peptides of bee venom phospholipase A2 induces specific T-cell anergy in patients allergic to bee venom. J Allergy Clin Immunol 101(6 Pt 1):747–754

Norman PS, Ohman JL, Long AA, Creticos PS, Gefter MA, Shaked Z et al (1996) Treatment of cat allergy with T-cell reactive peptides. Am J Respir Crit Care Med 154(6 Pt 1):1623–1628

Novak N, Bieber T, Katoh N (2001) Engagement of Fc epsilon RI on human monocytes induces the production of IL-10 and prevents their differentiation in dendritic cells. J Immunol 167(2):797–804

Oldfield WL, Kay AB, Larche M (2001) Allergen-derived T cell peptide-induced late asthmatic reactions precede the induction of antigen-specific hyporesponsiveness in atopic allergic asthmatic subjects. J Immunol 167(3):1734–1739

Oldfield WL, Larche M, Kay AB (2002) Effect of T-cell peptides derived from Fel d 1 on allergic reactions and cytokine production in patients sensitive to cats: a randomised controlled trial. Lancet 360(9326):47–53

Pene J, Desroches A, Paradis L, Lebel B, Farce M, Nicodemus CF et al (1998) Immunotherapy with Fel d 1 peptides decreases IL-4 release by peripheral blood T cells of patients allergic to cats. J Allergy Clin Immunol 102(4 Pt 1):571–578

Prakken BJ, van Der ZR, Anderton SM, van Kooten PJ, Kuis W, van Eden W (1997) Peptide-induced nasal tolerance for a mycobacterial heat shock protein 60 T cell epitope in rats suppresses both adjuvant arthritis and nonmicrobially induced experimental arthritis. Proc Natl Acad Sci USA 94(7):3284–3289

Reefer AJ, Carneiro RM, Custis NJ, Platts-Mills TA, Sung SS, Hammer J et al (2004) A role for IL-10-mediated HLA-DR7-restricted T cell-dependent events in development of the modified Th2 response to cat allergen. J Immunol 172(5):2763–2772

Santambrogio L, Sato AK, Fischer FR, Dorf ME, Stern LJ (1999a) Abundant empty class II MHC molecules on the surface of immature dendritic cells. Proc Natl Acad Sci USA 96(26):15050–15055

Santambrogio L, Sato AK, Carven GJ, Belyanskaya SL, Strominger JL, Stern LJ (1999b) Extracellular antigen processing and presentation by immature dendritic cells. Proc Natl Acad Sci USA 96(26):15056–15061

Simons FE, Imada M, Li Y, Watson WT, HayGlass KT (1996) Fel d 1 peptides: effect on skin tests and cytokine synthesis in cat-allergic human subjects. Int Immunol 8(12):1937–1945

Smith TR, Alexander C, Kay AB, Larche M, Robinson DS (2004) Cat allergen peptide immunotherapy reduces CD4 T cell responses to cat allergen but does not alter suppression by CD4 CD25 T cells: a double-blind placebo-controlled study. Allergy 59(10):1097–1101

Staines NA, Harper N, Ward FJ, Malmstrom V, Holmdahl R, Bansal S (1996) Mucosal tolerance and suppression of collagen-induced arthritis (CIA) induced by nasal inhalation of synthetic peptide 184-198 of bovine type II collagen (CII) expressing a dominant T cell epitope. Clin Exp Immunol 103(3):368–375

Steinman RM, Hawiger D, Nussenzweig MC (2003) Tolerogenic dendritic cells. Annu Rev Immunol 21:685–711.

Tarzi M, Klunker S, Texier C, Verhoef A, Stapel SO, Akdis C et al (2005) Induction of interleukin-10 and suppressor of cytokine signaling-3 gene expression following peptide immunotherapy. Clin Exp Allergy

Texier C, Pouvelle S, Busson M, Herve M, Charron D, Menez A et al (2000) HLA-DR restricted peptide candidates for bee venom immunotherapy. J Immunol 164(6):3177–3184

Tian J, Atkinson MA, Clare-Salzler M, Herschenfeld A, Forsthuber T, Lehmann PV et al (1996) Nasal administration of glutamate decarboxylase (GAD65) peptides induces Th2 responses and prevents murine insulin-dependent diabetes. J Exp Med 183(4):1561–1567

Verhoef A, Alexander C, Kay AB, Larche M (2005) T cell epitope immunotherapy induces a CD4(+) T cell population with regulatory activity. PLoS Med 2(3):e78

von Garnier C, Astori M, Kettner A, Dufour N, Heusser C, Corradin G et al (2000) Allergen-derived long peptide immunotherapy down-regulates specific IgE response and protects from anaphylaxis. Eur J Immunol 30(6):1638–1645

Wraith DC, Goldman M, Lambert PH (2003) Vaccination and autoimmune disease: what is the evidence? Lancet 362(9396):1659–1666

Wraith DC, Nicolson KS, Whitley NT (2004) Regulatory CD4(+) T cells and the control of autoimmune disease. Curr Opin Immunol 16(6):695–701

Allergen-Specific Immunotherapy: Towards Combination Vaccines for Allergic and Infectious Diseases

Johanna Edlmayr, Katarzyna Niespodziana, Margarete Focke-Tejkl, Birgit Linhart and Rudolf Valenta

Abstract IgE-mediated allergies affect more than 25% of the population. Allergen-specific immunotherapy (SIT) is an antigen-specific and disease-modifying form of treatment. It is based on the therapeutic administration of the disease-causing allergens to allergic patients. However, the fact that only allergen extracts of insufficient quality are currently available and the possible occurrence of side effects during treatment limit the broad use of SIT and prophylactic vaccination is has not yet been performed. In the last 20 years the DNA sequences of the most common allergens have been isolated and the corresponding allergens have been produced as recombinant allergens. Based on the progress made in the field of allergen characterization it is possible to improve the quality and safety of allergy vaccines and to develop new, more effective strategies for a broad application of SIT and even for prophylactic treatment. Here we discuss the development of combination vaccines for allergy and infectious diseases. This approach is based on the selection of allergen-derived peptides with reduced IgE- and T cell reactivity in order to minimize IgE- and T cell-mediated side effects as well as the potential of the vaccine to induce allergic sensitization. These peptides are fused by recombinant technology onto a viral carrier protein to obtain a combination vaccine which induces protective immunity against allergy and viral infections. The application of such combination vaccines for therapy and prophylaxis of allergy and infectious diseases is discussed.

J. Edlmayr · K. Niespodziana · B. Linhart · R. Valenta
Division of Immunopathology, Department of Pathophysiology and Allergy Research, Center for Pathophysiology, Infectiology and Immunology, Medical University of Vienna, Vienna, Austria

M. Focke-Tejkl · R. Valenta (✉)
Christian Doppler Laboratory for Allergy Research, Medical University of Vienna, AKH Ebene 3Q, Waehringer Guertel 18–20, 1090 Vienna, Austria
e-mail: rudolf.valenta@meduniwien.ac.at

Current Topics in Microbiology and Immunology (2011) 352: 121–140
DOI: 10.1007/82_2011_130

Published Online: 29 May 2011

Contents

1 Introduction

Allergen contact and allergic inflammation can occur in different target organs leading to mild (e.g., rhinoconjunctivitis), more severe (e.g., asthma), and systemic, life-threatening manifestations (e.g., anaphylactic shock). Mild respiratory allergy, for example, rhinitis, frequently progresses to asthma, a severe disabling respiratory form of allergy affecting the lung. Asthma is a chronic disease characterized by airway hyper-responsiveness, airway inflammation, airway remodeling and reversible airway obstruction. Patients with inadequately controlled severe persistent asthma are at a particularly high risk of exacerbations, hospitalization and death (Demoly and Bousquet 2006; Peters et al. 2006). In this context it should also be mentioned that asthma is triggered by a variety of other factors such as viral infections or pollutants (Holgate 2006; Bousquet et al. 2005).

Sensitization to allergens, i.e., the production of allergen-specific IgE antibodies, occurs in genetically predisposed individuals (i.e., atopic individuals) shortly after birth and can be modulated by a variety of environmental factors (Kulig et al. 1999; Niederberger et al. 2002; Platts-Mills 2005; Vercelli 2006; Garn and Renz 2007). Subsequent allergen contact strongly boosts the established secondary IgE response and clinical sensitivity in allergic patients (Yunginger and Gleich 1973; Henderson et al. 1975; Niederberger et al. 2007). Acute allergic inflammation is mainly due to the activation of mast cells and basophils by IgE-allergen immune complexes whereas T cells and eosinophils play an important role in chronic allergic inflammation (reviewed in Valenta 2002; Desreumaux and Capron 1996).

Mast cells and basophils bind allergen-specific IgE antibodies via the high affinity receptor for IgE, FcεRI, which can be cross-linked by allergens to release inflammatory mediators, pro-inflammatory cytokines and proteases (Bischoff 2007). These substances cause immediate allergic inflammation, tissue damage and attract inflammatory cells. Allergen contact also activates allergen-specific T cells to release pro-inflammatory cytokines leading to chronic allergic inflammation (Larche et al. 2003). The presentation of allergens to T cells can be facilitated by IgE bound to Fcε Receptors on the surface of antigen presenting cells (dendritic cells, monocytes) and B-cells or occur in an IgE-independent manner (van Neerven et al. 2006; Haselden et al. 1999; Campana et al. 2008).

Allergen-specific immunotherapy (SIT) is the only antigen-specific and disease-modifying treatment of allergy. It has been also demonstrated that SIT can prevent the progression of allergic rhinitis to asthma (Moller et al. 2002).

SIT is based on the administration of the disease-eliciting allergens (reviewed in Larche et al. 2006). This treatment has been developed exactly 100 years ago when Noon and later Freeman injected grass pollen extract into grass pollen allergic patients (Noon 1911; Freeman 1914). In the next chapter we review some milestones in the development of SIT.

2 Developments in the Field of Allergen-specific Immunotherapy

Reactions to different substances were described already in the antique, but Bostock was the first, who published in 1819 an official medical case report of hay fever, referring to his own personal experience. Wyman and especially Blackley identified pollen as source for allergens, demonstrated that pollen exposure can induce allergic reactions and measured pollen exposure (Bostock 1819; Wyman 1872; Blackley 1873). Hundred years ago it was not known that allergy is an immunologically-mediated disease but Noon injected pollen extracts into hay fever patients based on the hypothesis that they suffered from intoxication (Noon 1911).

Between 1913 and 1959 the idea was pursued that not only administration of pollen, but also bacterial vaccines may have beneficial effects on hay fever (Morrey 1913). In this context it was also reported that skin reactions and systemic reactions not only occurred on exposure to pollens and food, but also with bacterial products, such as tuberculin which led to the presumption that bacteria may cause allergic reactions (Walker and Adkinson 1917). Interestingly, a connection between respiratory tract infections and asthma or asthma exacerbations was already described 1932 (Cooke 1932). However, clinical trials with bacterial vaccines against asthma were not performed until 1955 and failed to be effective (Frankland et al. 1955; Johnstone 1957; Helander 1959).

SIT as introduced by Noon and Freeman continued to be a successful treatment also for other allergen sources. A first controlled immunotherapy trial was performed in 1954 and a first double-blind study in 1965. It could be shown that SIT resulted in fewer symptoms and lower medication scores compared to control groups (Frankland and Augustin 1954; Lowell and Franklin 1965).

The understanding of the mechanisms underlying allergy developed in parallel to the use of SIT. In an elegant experiment Prausnitz and Kuestner demonstrated in

1921 that allergen-specific sensitivity can be transferred to a non-allergic person by injection of serum from the allergic individual (Prausnitz and Kuestner 1921). This experiment indicated that serum from allergic patients contains allergen-specific factors, later termed reagins, which combine with a non-specific tissue component also present in healthy persons and then give rise to an allergic reaction induced by the allergen. It took more than 40 years until the serum factor could be isolated by K. and T. Ishizaka (1967) and was identified as immunoglobulin E through comparison with a myeloma protein discovered by Johansson and Bennich (1967). Based on the availability of the IgE myeloma the RAST test for measuring IgE antibodies in sera could be developed for the diagnosis of allergic patients (Wide et al. 1967).

Long before the characterization of "reaginic" IgE, i.e., in 1935, it could be demonstrated that patients receiving SIT developed antigen-specific serum factors (i.e., blocking IgG antibodies) that blocked allergic skin reactions (Cooke et al. 1935).

Loveless (1940) demonstrated that blocking antibodies compete with reagins for the binding sites on allergens and Lichtenstein et al. (1968) showed that the blocking antibodies belong to the IgG class.

Rocklin et al. (1980) proposed suppressor cells as another possible mechanism of SIT. They detected allergen-specific suppressor cells in ragweed allergic patients after injections with ragweed extract, but not before immunotherapy.

After introduction of the Th1/Th2 concept into human allergy (Paronchi et al. 1991) it was suggested that SIT may affect the Th1/Th2 balance (Secrist et al. 1993).

More recently the possibility has been discussed that SIT, or at least certain forms of SIT, may induce allergen-specific immune tolerance mediated through tolerogenic cytokines and possibly regulatory T cells (Akdis et al. 1998). The contribution of the various mechanisms (e.g., induction of blocking antibodies, affecting the Th2/Th1 balance and tolerogenic mechanisms) to efficacy of the various forms of SIT is a matter of intense investigation (Larche et al. 2006). However, many recent studies performed with purified allergens/recombinant allergens and recombinant hypoallergenic allergen derivatives speak for an important role of allergen-specific IgG antibodies in preventing allergen-induced inflammation and allergen-induced boosts of the allergic immune response (Valenta et al. 2010).

So far, the vast majority of immunotherapy studies and the analysis of these studies have been carried out with allergen extracts from natural sources. However, these extracts are often of poor quality. For example, the allergen concentrations vary between different extract preparations and contain biologic active allergens in different concentrations as well as non-allergenic components (Focke et al. 2008, 2009; Curin et al. 2010; Brunetto et al. 2010). The heterogeneity of allergen extracts certainly represents a major bottleneck limiting the broad use of SIT. It has hampered the analysis of the mechanisms of SIT and is responsible for the sometimes poor clinical efficacy.

The efforts to improve the quality of allergen extracts have already started early. For example, Stull et al. (1933) worked on standardization of allergen batches and developed a measurement of protein nitrogen units for the assessment of allergenic activity. King and Norman started to isolate the major allergen fractions of ragweed pollen in 1962 (King and Norman 1962). However, despite all standardization efforts which later involved measurements of allergenic activity, IgE binding capacity and the measurement of major allergens in the extracts the fact remains that the composition of allergen extracts cannot be influenced by the manufacturer.

The administration of allergen extracts to patients in the course of SIT can cause side effects which may be mild and local but also severe, systemic and life-threatening (Mellerup et al. 2000).

Therefore several efforts for the reduction of allergenic side effects have been made. Seventy years ago aluminium-hydroxide-adsorbed allergen extracts were introduced for depot vaccination, showing improved immune stimulatory as well as reduced anaphylactic properties (Zoss et al. 1937). Already in 1969 allergen-derived peptides were used for immunotherapy. In fact, Malley and Perlman used the low-molecular-weight fragment of allergen extracts for SIT and induced blocking antibodies (Malley and Perlman 1969). During 1970 and 1980 further attempts for the reduction of side effects were made by chemical modification of allergens (Marsh et al. 1970; Lee and Sehon 1978).

In its beginning, SIT had been typically administered by subcutaneous injection. In order to facilitate SIT and make it more convenient many attempts have been made to administer SIT via other routes. Already in 1921 and 1922 MacKenzie, Caulfield and Touart tried to desensitize allergic patients by nasal, oral and throat administration of pollen in form of sprays and ointments (MacKenzie 1922; Caulfield 1922; Touart 1922). However, Feinberg et al. demonstrated in a multicenter placebo-controlled study that the oral application of high doses of ragweed pollen lacked efficacy (Feinberg 1940). Further attempts to give oral immunotherapy started in the early 1970s with controversial results until today (Laetsch and Wuthrich 1973; Urbanek et al. 1990; Mosbech et al. 1987; Scadding and Brostoff 1986). Until today several thousand individuals have been treated in various clinical studies with sublingual immunotherapy (SLIT) but the mechanisms of this treatment are still unknown. There are even studies demonstrating that SLIT induces strong boosts of allergen-specific IgE production (Durham et al. 2006). Generally, there is a lack of studies which have investigated effects of SLIT on objective outcome parameters such as allergen-specific skin or target organ sensitivity. Yet there is evidence from meta-analysis for clinical efficacy of SLIT but these effects seem to be much less than those obtained by subcutaneous SIT, although this is difficult to assess because only few studies comparing subcutaneous SIT and SLIT have been carried out (Radulovic et al. 2010).

3 The Impact of Recombinant Allergens on SIT

With the introduction of recombinant DNA technology into the field of allergen characterization it has become possible to reveal the sequences and structures of the most common allergens. A large number of the most important disease-eliciting allergens have been characterized down to the molecular level and recombinant allergens mimicking the epitope complexity of natural allergen extracts have been produced. According to the allergen-encoding DNA sequence, recombinant allergens can be produced as highly pure proteins and used for diagnostic and therapeutic purposes (Valenta et al. 2010).

3.1 Recombinant Wildtype Allergens

The term "recombinant wildtype allergen" describes a recombinant allergen, which mimics the allergenic properties of the natural allergen derived from the natural allergen source. It contains the relevant IgE- and T cell epitopes of the natural allergen and hence can be used for diagnosis and therapy similar to allergen extracts. Advantages of recombinant allergens over extracts are that they represent well defined and highly pure proteins. When used for SIT, recombinant allergens are expected to induce similar effects as natural allergens which has indeed been shown in first immunotherapy studies using purified recombinant grass pollen allergens (Jutel et al. 2005). In a SIT trial in 2006 birch pollen allergic patients received recombinant Bet v 1a, purified natural Bet v 1 and birch pollen extract. This study showed in a direct comparison that a single recombinant allergen is as effective as treatment with the natural extract (Pauli et al. 2008).

Recombinant wildtype allergens carry the IgE and T cell epitopes of the corresponding natural allergen and upon SIT induce allergen-specific IgG blocking antibodies and depending on the dose, route and adjuvant may induce Th1 immune responses. Due to the presence of allergen-specific T cell epitopes, recombinant wildtype allergens could in principle induce T cell tolerance, which may also depend on the dose, mode and route of application. Disadvantages of recombinant wildtype allergens are that they can induce both, IgE as well as T cell-mediated side effects and that their administration may induce new sensitizations or boost an existing allergen-specific IgE response.

The first allergens made by recombinant DNA technology were Dol m V (major allergen of white-face hornet venom), Der p 1 (major house dust mite allergen) and Bet v 1 (major allergen of birch pollen) published in the late 1980's (Fang et al. 1988; Breiteneder et al. 1989; Chua et al. 1988).

Recombinant allergens were first used for allergy diagnosis in 1991. Valenta et al. tested birch pollen allergic patients' sera for Bet v 1- and Bet v 2-specific reactivity and revealed a similar IgE-binding pattern as with natural allergens (Valenta et al. 1991).

The first animal models and *in vivo* applications in patients with recombinant allergens were performed 1992 and 1994 (Sehon and Mohapatra 1992; Moser et al. 1994). Sehon and Mohapatra induced IgE antibodies specific for recombinant grass pollen antigens from Poa pratensis in mice. First skin test studies demonstrating the biological equivalence of recombinant and natural allergens from

Aspergillus and house dust mites were carried out in 1994 (Moser et al. 1994; Lynch et al. 1994).

Today cDNAs coding for the most common allergens have been isolated and the corresponding recombinant allergens are available for research purposes, diagnosis and treatment (reviewed in Valenta et al. 2010).

3.2 Hypoallergenic Allergen Derivatives

Recombinant allergens that resemble natural wild type allergens contain all relevant IgE epitopes and therefore retain the risk of inducing IgE-mediated side effects. Therefore modifications have been introduced to generate hypoallergenic allergen derivatives. These new molecules should show abolished or substantially reduced IgE-binding activity while retaining T cell reactivity and immunogenicity. Several strategies for the modification of an allergen were developed (Valenta 2002).

In fact, the first immunotherapy trial with recombinant molecules has been performed with genetically modified hypoallergenic derivatives of the major birch pollen allergen, Bet v 1 ten years ago (Niederberger 2004). Patients received either recombinant Bet v 1 fragments or a recombinant trimer of Bet v 1. Although patients had received only one treatment course they developed a robust IgG (IgG1, IgG2, IgG4) antibody response against natural Bet v 1, Bet v 1-related pollen allergens from alder and hazels and food allergens (apple, carrot, celery). The concept of recombinant hypoallergens has meanwhile been successfully evaluated in clinical immunotherapy trials for the treatment of birch pollen allergy up to phase III trials (Klimek et al. 2005; Rak 2009; Valenta et al. 2011).

3.3 Recombinant Hybrid Molecules

Very often certain allergens have low immunogenicity and there are allergen sources containing several allergens which need to be included in the vaccine. In order to address the problem hybrid allergens were generated by sequential fusion of cDNAs encoding for different allergens. As it has been shown for grass pollen allergy it is possible to produce recombinant hybrid molecules consisting of the most relevant allergens either as wild type allergens or as hypoallergenic allergen derivatives and thus to combine the relevant epitopes in one protein with increased immunogenicity (Linhart et al. 2002, 2005, 2008).

3.4 DNA Vaccines

Hsu et al. and Raz et al. published the first papers using DNA vaccines for the treatment of allergy in experimental animal models. The data of their studies performed in mice demonstrated that this approach prevents the induction of IgE synthesis, IL-4 and IL-5 production as well as histamine release (Hsu et al. 1996; Raz et al. 1996).

3.5 Allergen Conjugates

Another strategy concerns immunostimulation using allergen conjugates where allergen components are fused to a foreign molecule. For example, synthetic DNA sequences that contain CpG motifs have been linked to allergens to generate immunostimulatory conjugates. Treatment of allergic patients with the major ragweed allergen in a placebo-controlled study resulted in redirection of ragweed-specific Th2 responses towards Th1 responses (Simons et al. 2004). These responses were characterized by increased production of INF-γ and decreased production of IL-5. The injection of the CpG-Amb a 1 fusion product induced no clinically significant systemic or local allergic reactions and showed promising results in an immunotherapy trial (Creticos et al. 2006).

Another conjugated product with immunostimulatory activity was developed by Bohle et al. In this study a fusion protein consisting of Bet v 1 and the bacterial cell surface protein SbsC was recombinantly produced and displayed reduced histamine-releasing capacity. Basophils of Allergic patients T cells exposed to rSbsC-Bet v 1 produced INF-γ and IL-10, but no IL-5 (Bohle et al. 2004). A reduction of allergenic activity and increase in immunogenicity was observed in murine models when the major cat allergen, Fel d 1 was conjugated to viral particles (Schmitz et al. 2009).

3.6 T Cell Epitope Peptides

A completely different strategy, for decreasing IgE-mediated side effects which is based on the administration of allergen-derived T cell-reactive peptides. Peptides are short in length and have a linear structure, which lead to a reduced ability to cross-link mast cell-and basophil-bound IgE and are therefore candidates for safe SIT. The mechanism behind the reduction of allergy symptoms using T-cell epitope containing peptides for SIT is the ability of the peptides to induce immunologic tolerance. Clinical trials using peptide immunotherapy have been mainly performed for cat and venom allergy (Ali and Larche 2005; Norman et al. 1996). T-cell epitope derived peptide immunotherapy with reduced IgE-mediated side effects, but it was reported that T cell epitope peptides of the major cat allergen, Fel d 1, induced asthma and bronchial hyper reactivity several hours after intracutaneous injection and this effect is T cell-mediated and MHC-restricted (Haselden et al. 1999).

These results indicate that the removal of IgE-reactivity diminishes IgE-mediated side effects but late phase side effects are common so attempts are currently being made to reduce them by adequate dosing.

3.7 *Allergen-Derived Peptides Lacking Allergenic Activity to Induce Allergen-Specific Blocking IgG Antibodies*

Long before the discovery of IgE antibodies it has been demonstrated that SIT induces allergen-specific IgG antibodies which inhibit binding of allergic patients IgE to the allergen (i.e., blocking antibodies) (Cooke et al. 1935; Loveless 1940). Several recent studies have been performed using well defined systems based on purified allergens and epitopes confirming that the induction of allergen-specific blocking antibodies is a major mechanism for the efficacy of SIT (reviewed in Larche et al. 2006; Valenta et al. 2010, 2004). Today we know that blocking IgG not only inhibits allergen-induced mast cell and basophil activation and thus immediate symptoms of allergy but also IgE-facilitated allergen presentation to T cells and thus reduces chronic allergic inflammation. Moreover, allergen-specific blocking IgG inhibits boosts of allergen-specific IgE production by capturing allergens and thus decreases allergen-specific IgE, a mechanisms which may be important for the long-lasting effects of SIT. We also know now that IgE antibodies mainly recognize conformational epitopes on allergens which require folded allergens with intact three-dimensional structure (Valenta et al. 2010). The latter has been recently visualized by the solution of the three-dimensional structures of complexes consisting of allergens and the corresponding patients IgE antibodies (Niemi et al. 2007; Padavattan et al. 2009).

It is therefore possible to engineer allergy vaccines based on allergen derivatives lacking fold and conformational IgE epitopes or in which amino acids necessary for IgE recognition have been altered (i.e., recombinant hypoallergenic allergen derivatives) (Valenta 2002). These molecules have been successfully used in immunotherapy trials and showed a lack of IgE-mediated side effects (Niederberger 2004; Klimek et al. 2005; Rak 2009; Purohit et al. 2008). However, since hypoallergenic allergen derivatives still contain allergen-specific T cell epitopes, these vaccines can still induce T cell-mediated side effects such as vaccines based on non-IgE-reactive peptides containing T cell epitopes (Haselden et al. 1999; Campana et al. 2008; Purohit et al. 2008).

Several years ago, Focke et al., have developed an approach for allergy vaccines inducing blocking antibodies using peptides derived from surface exposed areas and thus IgE recognition sites of allergens which lacked structure and hence IgE-reactivity (Focke et al. 2001, 2004). They showed that one or few peptides are sufficient to focus blocking IgG antibodies toward IgE binding sites on allergens. To induce peptide-specific and thus allergen-specific IgG antibodies they used foreign (i.e., non allergen-derived) carrier molecules such as KLH. Following the hapten carrier principle described by the Nobel laureate Benacerraf robust IgG responses against the peptide and antigens containing the peptides can be obtained using T cell help from the carrier (Siskind et al. 1966). The big advantage of the use of allergen-derived peptides lacking allergenic activity for the induction of allergen-specific blocking antibodies is that by choosing suitable peptides a large portion of allergen-sequences containing allergen-specific T cell epitopes can be eliminated so that these vaccines hold promise of not inducing T cell-mediated side effects (Focke et al. 2010). There is more and more data accumulating that suitable peptides can be identified for the most common allergens (e.g., grass pollen, birch pollen, house dust mites, olive pollen, cat) (Focke et al. 2001, 2004; Kundig et al. 2006; Twaroch et al. 2011; Niespodziana et al. 2011) and that these vaccines also have strongly reduced allergenicity i.e., they induce no or low allergic sensitization to the corresponding allergens and thus may be useful not only for therapeutic but also for prophylactic allergy vaccination.

Kündig et al. used the peptide approach in a phase I trial using a synthetic 16-amino-acid sequence of the allergen house dust mite Der p 1 which was chemically coupled to "virus-like particles", in fact to the bacteriophage Qbeta protein (Kundig et al. 2006). The vaccine induced IgG antibodies against Der p 1 and the virus-like particle and was well tolerated in healthy adults.

Since chemical coupling represents a poorly reproducible and cumbersome technology which is not well suited for vaccine production according to good manufacture practice (GMP) standards it is desirable to directly produce recombinant fusion proteins consisting of allergen-derived peptides lacking allergic activity and suitable carrier molecules which are safe and eventually foster a beneficial type of immune response.

4 Combination Vaccine against Allergies and Infectious Diseases

In search of suitable carrier molecules for the production of recombinant fusion proteins containing allergen-derived peptides without allergenic activity we considered pathogen-derived proteins because they may offer several advantages (Fig. 1). First, they may offer strong T cell help for robust IgG antibody production and thus have almost adjuvant-like activity, eventually twisting the resulting immune response away from the Th2 bias. Second, the pathogen-derived carrier proteins may induce anti-pathogen immunity and hence be useful for the prevention of infectious diseases (Fig. 2). Finally, it may be possible to use pathogen-derived molecules which have a proven track record of being safe vaccines in humans. In fact, vaccination against pathogens, in particular against viruses, bacteria and bacterial toxins is routinely applied in children for prophylactic purposes. In a first proof of principle study we have therefore expressed a fusion protein consisting of the capsid protein VP1 of human rhinoviruses and a peptide

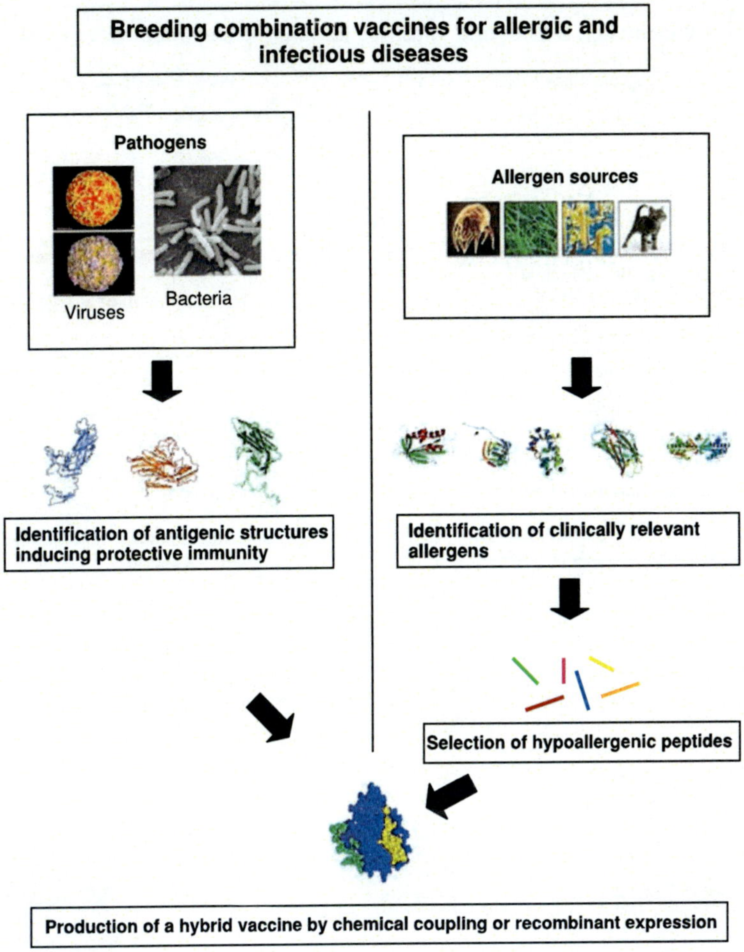

Fig. 1 Breeding combination vaccines for allergic and infectious diseases

derived from the major timothy grass pollen allergen, Phl p 1 (Edlmayr et al. 2009). The intention was to design an allergy vaccine which should not induce IgE- or T cell-mediated side effects and which may induce a protective effect against rhinovirus infections which are known as a major cause of asthma exacerbations (Holgate 2006). The rationale for selecting the viral protein VP1 was that it is involved in the interaction of the virus with ICAM 1 on epithelial cells (Greve et al. 1989). It was thus hoped that anti-VP1 antibodies would prevent the infection of epithelial cells by human rhinovirus. A recombinant fusion protein consisting of VP1 and a non-allergenic peptide of the major timothy grass pollen allergen Phl p 1 was made (Edlmayr et al. 2009). It was demonstrated that this fusion protein lacked IgE- or T-cell reactivity, but induced Phl p 1 specific blocking antibodies in mice and rabbits which inhibited allergic patients' IgE binding to the complete Phl

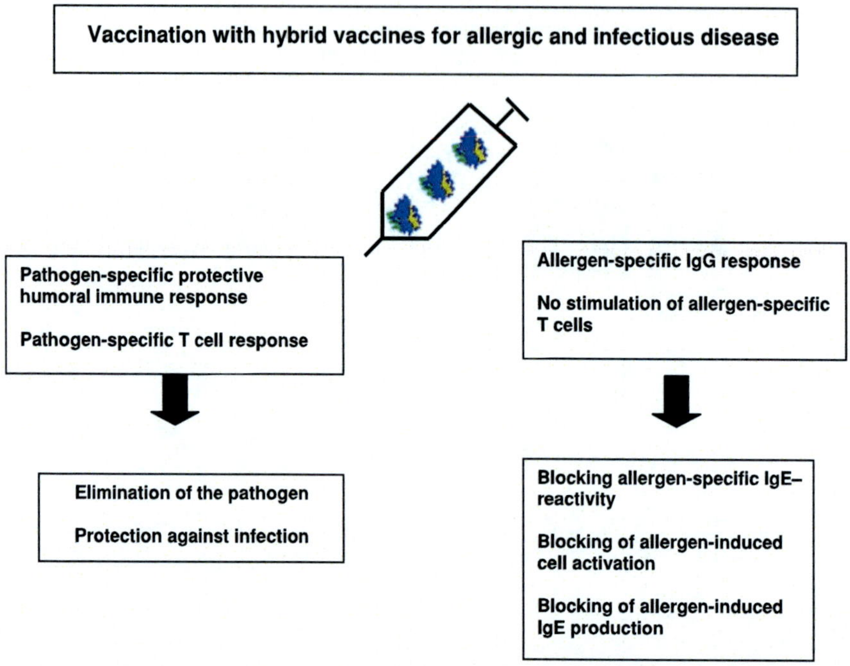

Fig. 2 Vaccination with hybrid vaccines for allergic and infectious disease

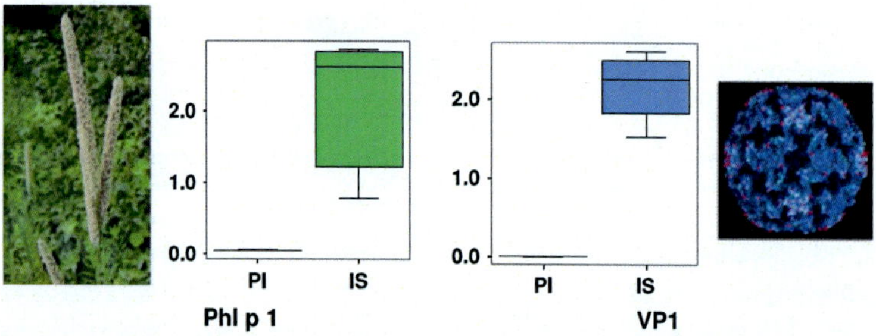

Fig. 3 Immune responses of immunized mice. Groups of mice were immunized with Phl p 1 (*left*) and VP1 (*right*). Serum samples were taken on the day of the first immunization (PI) and in three weeks interval. The immune sera (IS) were taken after three injections (*x-axis*). Phl p 1-specific IgG1 and VP1-specific titers were measured by ELISA and are expressed as optical value on the *y-axis*. The optical value corresponds to the level of IgG1 antibody in the mouse sera. The results are shown as *box plots* where 50% of the values are within the boxes and non-outliers between the bars. The lines within the boxes indicate the median values. Left: pictures of a meadow with timothy grass (*Phleum pratense*) right: rhinovirus image

p 1 allergen (Figs. 3, 4). It also blocked Phl p 1-induced immediate allergic inflammation as demonstrated by the inhibition of allergic patients' basophil degranulation. The VP1-based grass pollen vaccine induced in mice mainly

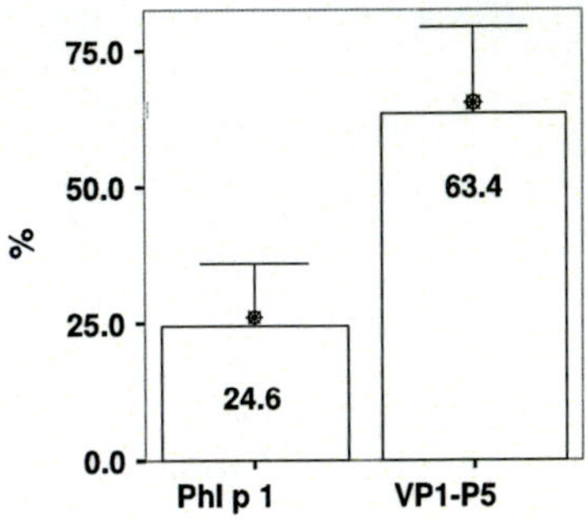

Fig. 4 Inhibition of grass pollen allergic patients IgE binding to Phl p 1 with rabbit antibodies against Phl p 1 and VP1-P5. Mean of percent inhibition of patient's ($n = 19$) IgE binding to Phl p 1 by preincubation with antisera against Phl p 1 or VP1-P5 (*x-axis*). The percent inhibition is shown at the *y-axis*

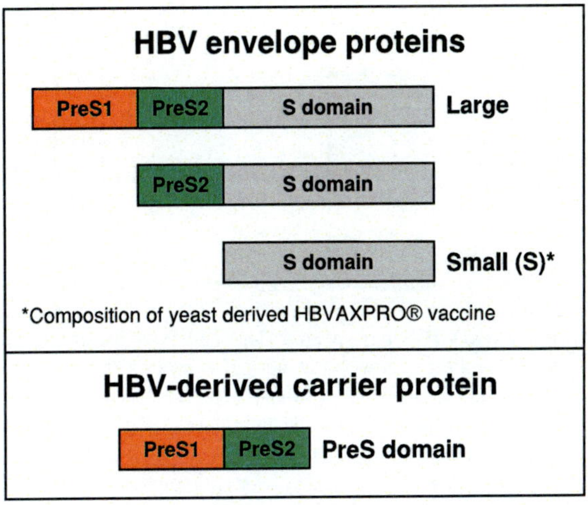

Fig. 5 Representation of the HBV envelope proteins and HBV-derived carrier protein. HBV envelope is composed of three related surface proteins known as large (L), middle (M) and small (S). These three proteins are products of the PreS1, PreS2 and S regions of the *env* gene. The small (S) envelope protein is widely and safely used worldwide for hepatitis B vaccination

VP1-specific T cell responses that shifted the Th2 response toward a mixed T_H1/T_H2 response. The resulting IgG subclasses were predominantly IgG1, but also IgG2a/b antibodies in mice vaccinated with the fusion protein.

In addition, the VP1 carrier induced IgG antibodies which prevented infection of epithelial cells against infection by rhinovirus and exhibited an unexpected broad cross-neutralization of several rhinovirus strains (Edlmayr et al. 2011).

Using a similar approach Niespodziana et al. produced a non-allergenic peptide vaccine consisting of the hepatitis PreS domain (Fig. 5) fused to non-allergenic peptides of the major cat allergen Fel d 1 and showed that this vaccine induced strong allergen-specific IgG responses which inhibited allergic patients IgE binding to Fel d 1 (Figs. 6, 7) (Niespodziana et al. 2011). The PreS fusion proteins could be expressed in large amounts in *Escherichia coli* under well standardized conditions and are attractive allergy vaccine candidates because PreS has been used safely for vaccination of newborns and children in clinical trials (Schumann et al. 2007).

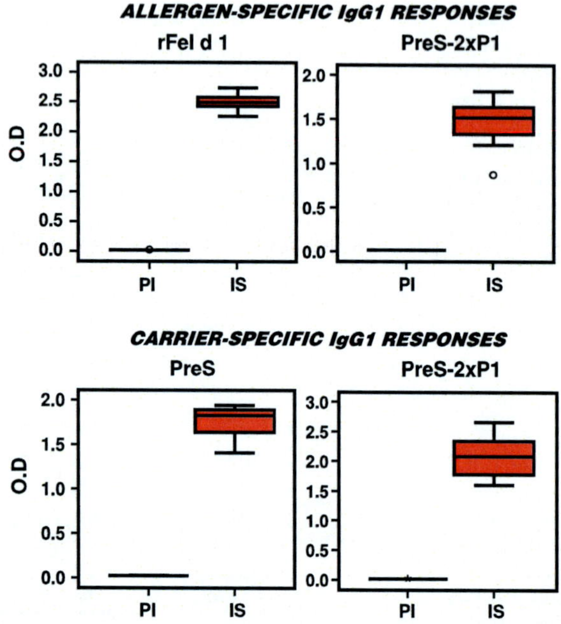

Fig. 6 Allergen-specific and carrier-specific IgG_1 responses in mice. Groups of mice were immunized subcutaneously with rFel d 1, PreS and PreS-2xP1 (*top of the boxes*). Serum samples were taken on the day before the first immunization (PI) and after the third injection (IS) (*x-axis*). rFel d 1-specific (*top*) and PreS-specific (*bottom*) IgG_1 titers were determined by ELISA and are expressed as optical values on the *y-axis*. The optical value corresponds to the level of IgG_1 antibody in mouse sera. The results are shown as *box plots* where 50% of the values are within the boxes and non-outliers between the bars. The line within the *boxes* indicates the median values

Fig. 7 Inhibition of cat allergic patients' IgE binding to rFel d 1 by anti-rFel d 1 and anti-PreS-P1-P5 rabbit IgG antibodies. Inhibitions of cat allergic patients' IgE binding to rFel d 1 by rabbit antisera (*x-axis*) are expressed as percentages of inhibition using preimmune sera as a reference. The mean percent inhibition for 26 patients is shown at the *y-axis*

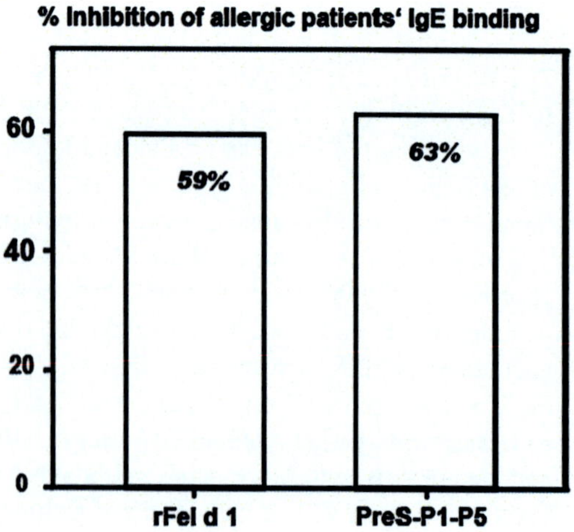

At present the preclinical evaluation of a grass pollen vaccine based on non-allergenic peptides of the four major timothy grass pollen allergens, Phl p 1, Phl p 2, Phl p 5 and Phl p 6, has been performed and safety skin tests and first safety and dose-finding immunotherapy trials in allergic patients are scheduled for 2011. According to preclinical testing, the new generation of non-allergenic vaccines based on fusion proteins consisting of viral carrier proteins and allergen-derived peptides has similar properties as the recombinant hypoallergenic allergen derivatives but should not induce IgE or T cell-mediated side effects. It is thus hoped that this new generation of vaccines will break the ground for the broad, convenient (i.e., only few administrations) and side effect-free applicability of SIT and eventually be useful for prophylactic allergy vaccination.

References

Akdis CA, Blesken T, Akdis M, Wünthrich B, Blaser K (1998) Role of interleukin 10 in specific immunotherapy. J Clin Invest 102:98–106

Ali FR, Larche M (2005) Peptide-based immunotherapy: a novel strategy for allergic disease. Expert Rev Vaccines 4:881–889

Bischoff SC (2007) Role of mast cells in allergic and non-allergic immune responses: comparison of human and murine data. Nat Rev Immunol 7:93–104

Blackley CH (1873) Experimental researches on the causes and nature of catarrhus aestivus (hay-fever or hay-asthma). Baillière, Tindall & Cox, London

Bohle B, Breitwieser A, Zwolfer B, Jahn-Schmid B, Sara M, Sleytr UB, Ebner C (2004) A novel approach to specific allergy treatment: the recombinant fusion protein of a bacterial cell surface (S-layer) protein and the major birch pollen allergen Bet v 1 (rSbsC-Bet v 1) combines reduced allergenicity with immunomodulating capacity. J Immunol 172:6642–6648

Bostock J (1819) Case of periodical affections of the eyes and chest. Med Chir Trans 10:161

Bousquet J, Bousquet PJ, Godard P, Daures JP (2005) The public health implications of asthma. Bull World Health Organ 83:548–554

Breiteneder H, Pettenburger K, Bito A, Valenta R, Kraft D, Rumpold H, Scheiner O, Breitenbach M (1989) The gene coding for the major birch pollen allergen Betv1, is highly homologous to a pea disease resistance response gene. Embo J 8:1935–1938

Brunetto B, Tinghino R, Braschi MC, Antonicelli L, Pini C, Lacovacci P (2010) Characterization and comparison of commercially available mite extracts for in vivo diagnosis. Allergy 65:184–190

Campana R, Mothes N, Rauter I, Vrtala S, Reininger R, Focke-Tejkl M, Lupinek C, Balic N, Spitzauer S, Valenta R (2008) Non-IgE-mediated chronic allergic skin inflammation revealed with rBet v 1 fragments. J Allergy Clin Immunol 121:528–530

Caulfield AHW (1922) Desensitization of hay fever patients by injection and local application. J Am Med Assoc 79:125

Chua KY, Stewart GA, Thomas WR, Simpson RJ, Dilworth RJ, Plozza TM, Turner KJ (1988) Sequence analysis of cDNA coding for a major house dust mite allergen, Der p 1. Homology with cysteine proteases. J Exp Med 167:175–182

Cooke RA (1932) Infective asthma: indication of its allergic nature. Am J Med Sci 183:309

Cooke RA, Barnard SH, Hrbald AT, Stull A (1935) Serological evidence of immunity with co-existing sensitisation in a type-of human allergy, hay fever. J Exp Med 62:733–750

Creticos PS, Schroeder JT, Hamilton RG, Balcer-Whaley SL, Khattignavong AP, Lindblad R, Li H, Coffman R, Seyfert V, Eiden JJ, Broide D (2006) Immunotherapy with a ragweed-toll-like receptor 9 agonist vaccine for allergic rhinitis. N Engl J Med 355:1445–1455

Curin M, Reininger R, Swoboda I, Focke M, Valenta R, Spitzauer S (2010) Skin prick test extracts for dog allergy diagnosis show considerable variations regarding the content of major and minor dog allergens. Int Arch Allergy Immunol 154:258–263

Demoly P, Bousquet J (2006) The relation between asthma and allergic rhinitis. Lancet 368:711–713

Desreumaux, P, Capron M (1996) Eosinophils in allergic reactions. Curr Opin Immunol 8: 790–795

Durham SR, Yang WH, Pedersen MR, Johansen N, Rak S (2006) Sublingual immunotherapy with once-daily grass allergen tablets: a randomized controlled trial in seasonal allergic rhinoconjuncivitis. J Allergy Clin Immunol 117:802–809

Edlmayr J, Niespodziana K, Linhart B, Focke-Tejkl M, Westritschnig K, Scheiblhofer S, Stoecklinger A, Kneidinger M, Valent P, Campana R, Thalhamer J, Popow-Kraupp T, Valenta R (2009) A combination vaccine for allergy and rhinovirus infections based on rhinovirus-derived surface protein VP1 and a nonallergenic peptide of the major timothy grass pollen allergen Phl p 1. J Immunol 182:6298–6306

Edlmayr J, Niespodziana K, Popow-Kraupp T, Krzyzanek V, Focke-Tejkl M, Blaas D, Grote M, Valenta R (2011) Antibodies induced with recombinant VP1 from Human rhinovirus exhibit cross-neutralization. Eur Respir J 37:44–52

Fang KS, Vitale M, Fehlner P, King TP (1988) cDNA cloning and primary structure of a white-face hornet venom allergen, antigen 5. Proc Natl Acad Sci USA 85:895–899

Feinberg SM (1940) Oral pollen therapy in ragweed pollinosis. J Am Med Assoc 115:231

Focke M, Mahler V, Ball T, Sperr WR, Majlesi Y, Valent P, Kraft D, Valenta R (2001) Nonanaphylactic synthetic peptides derived from B cell epitopes of the major grass pollen allergen, Phl p 1, for allergy vaccination. Faseb J 15:2042–2044

Focke M, Linhart B, Hartl A, Wiedermann U, Sperr WR, Valent P, Thalhamer J, Kraft D, Valenta R (2004) Non-anaphylactic surface-exposed peptides of the major birch pollen allergen, Bet v 1, for preventive vaccination. Clin Exp Allergy 34:1525–1533

Focke M, Marth K, Flicker S, Valenta R (2008) Heterogeneity of commercial timothy grass pollen extracts. Clin Exp Allergy 38:1400–1408

Focke M, Marth K, Valenta R (2009) Molecular composition and biological activity of commercial birch pollen allergen extracts. Eur J Clin Invest 39:429–436

Focke M, Swoboda I, Marth K, Valenta R (2010) Developments in allergen-specific immunotherapy: from allergen extracts to allergy vaccines bypassing allergen-specific immunoglobulin E and T cell reactivity. Clin Exp Allergy 40:385–397

Frankland AW, Augustin R (1954) Prophylaxis of summer hay-fever and asthma: a controlled trial comparing crude grass-pollen extracts with the isolated main protein component. Lancet 266:1055–1057

Frankland AW, Hughes WH, Gorrill RH (1955) Autogenous bacterial vaccines in treatment of asthma. Br Med J 2:941–944

Freeman J (1914) Vaccination against hay fever; report of results during the last three years Lancet 1:1178

Garn H, Renz H (2007) Epidemiological and immunological evidence for the hygiene hypothesis. Immunobiology 212:441–452

Greve JM, Davis G, Meyer AM (1989) The major human rhinovirus receptor is ICAM-1. Cell 56: 839–847

Haselden BM, Kay AB, Larche M (1999) Immunoglobulin E-independent major histocompatibility complex-restricted T cell peptide epitope-induced late asthmatic reactions. J Exp Med 189:1885–1894

Helander E (1959) Bacterial vaccines in the treatment of bronchial asthma. Acta Allergy 13:47

Henderson LL, Larson JB, Gleich GJ (1975) Maximal rise in IgE antibody following ragweed pollination season. J Allergy Clin Immunol 55:10–15

Holgate ST (2006) Rhinoviruses in the pathogenesis of asthma: the bronchial epithelium as a major disease target. J Allergy Clin Immunol 118:587–590

Hsu CH, Chua KY, Tao MH, Lai YL, Wu HD, Huang SK, Hsieh KH (1996) Immunoprophylaxis of allergen-induced immunoglobulin E synthesis and airway hyperresponsiveness in vivo by genetic immunization. Nat Med 2:540–544

Ishizaka K, Ishizaka T (1967) Identification of gamma-E-antibodies as a carrier of reaginic activity. J Immunol 99:1187–1198

Johansson SG, Bennich H (1967) Immunological studies of an atypical (myeloma) immunoglobulin. Immunology 13:381–384

Johnstone DE (1957) Study of the value of bacterial vaccines in the treatment of bronchial asthma associated with respiratory infections. Am J Dis Child 94:1

Jutel M, Jaeger L, Suck R, Meyer H, Fiebig H, Cromwell O (2005) Allergen-specific immunotherapy with recombinant grass pollen allergens. J Allergy Clin Immunol 116:608–613

King TP, Norman PS (1962) Isolation studies of allergens from ragweed pollen. Biochemistry 1:709

Klimek L, Bachert C, Doemer C, Meyer H, Narkus A (2005) Specific immunotherapy with recombinant birch pollen allergen rBet v 1-FV is clinically efficacious. Allergy Clin Immunol Int (Suppl 1):15

Kulig M, Bergmann R, Klettke U, Wahn V, Tacke U, Wahn U (1999) Natural course of sensitization to food and inhalant allergens during the first 6 years of life. J Allergy Clin Immunol 103:1173–1179

Kundig TM, Senti G, Schnetzler G, Wolf C, Prinz Vavricka BM, Fulurija A, Hennecke F, Sladko K, Jennings GT, Bachmann MF (2006) Der p 1 peptide on virus-like particles is safe and highly immunogenic in healthy adults. J Allergy Clin Immunol 117:1470–1476

Laetsch C, Wuthrich B (1973) Peroral desensitization of inhalation allergies in childhood: treatment results. Schweiz Med Wochenschr 103:342–347

Larche M, Robinson DS, Kay AB (2003) The role of T lymphocytes in the pathogenesis of asthma. J Allergy Clin Immunol 111:450–463, quiz 464

Larche M, Akdis CA, Valenta R (2006) Immunological mechanisms of allergen-specific immunotherapy. Nat Rev Immunol 6:761–771

Lee WY, Sehon AH (1978) Suppression of reaginic antibodies with modified allergens. I. Reduction in allergenicity of protein allergens by conjugation to polyethylene glycol. Int Arch Allergy Appl Immunol 56:159–170

Lichtenstein LM, Holtzman NA, Burnett LS (1968) A quantitative in vitro study of the chromatographic distribution and immunoglobulin characteristics of human blocking antibody. J Immunol 101:317–324

Linhart B, Jahn-Schmid B, Verdino P, Keller W, Ebner C, Kraft D, Valenta R (2002) Combination vaccines for the treatment of grass pollen allergy consisting of genetically engineered hybrid molecules with increased immunogenicity. Faseb J 16:1301–1303

Linhart B, Hartl A, Jahn-Schmid B, Verdino P, Keller W, Krauth MT, Valent P, Horak F, Wiedermann U, Thalhamer J, Ebner C, Kraft D, Valenta R (2005) A hybrid molecule resembling the epitope spectrum of grass pollen for allergy vaccination. J Allergy Clin Immunol 115:1010–1016

Linhart B, Mothes-Luksch N, Vrtala S, Kneidinger M, Valent P, Valenta R (2008) A hypoallergenic hybrid molecule with increased immunogenicity consisting of derivatives of the major grass pollen allergens, Phl p 2 and Phl p 6. Biol chem 389:925–933

Loveless MH (1940) Immunological studies of pollenosis. IV. The presence of two antibodies related to the same pollen antigen in the serum of treated hay fever patients. J Immunol 38:20–50

Lowell FC, Franklin W (1965) A double-blind study of the effectiveness and specificity of injecton therapy in ragweed hay fever. N Engl J Med 273:675–679

Lynch NR, Thomas WR, Chua Y, Garcia N, Di Prisco MC, Lopez R (1994) In vivo biological activity of recombinant Der p II allergen of house-dust mite. Int Arch Allergy Immunol 105:70–74

MacKenzie GM (1922) Desensitzation of hay fever patients by specific local application. J Am Med Assoc 78:787

Malley A, Perlman F (1969) Induction of both reaginic and blocking antibodies with a low molecular weight fraction of timothy pollen extract. J Allergy 43:59–64

Marsh DG, Lichtenstein LM, Campbell DH (1970) Studies on "allergoids" prepared from naturally occurring allergens. I. Assay of allergenicity and antigenicity of formalinized rye group I component. Immunology 18:705–722

Mellerup MT, Hahn GW, Poulsen LK, Malling H (2000) Safety of allergen specific immunotherapy. Relation between dosage regimen, allergen extract, disease and systemic side-effects during induction treatment. Clin Exp Allergy 30:1423–1429

Moller C, Dreborg S, Ferdousi HA, Halken S, Host A, Jacobsen L, Koivikko A, Koller DY, Niggemann B, Norberg LA, Urbanek R, Valovirta E, Wahn U (2002) Pollen immunotherapy reduces the development of asthma in children with seasonal rhinoconjunctivitis (the PAT-study). J Allergy Clin Immunol 109:251–256

Morrey CB (1913) Vaccination with mixed cultures from the nose in hay fever. J Am Med Assoc 61:1806

Mosbech H, Dreborg S, Madsen F, Ohlsson H, Stahl Skov P, Taudorf E, Weeke B (1987) High dose grass pollen tablets used for hyposensitization in hay fever patients. A one-year double blind placebo-controlled study. Allergy 42:451–455

Moser M, Crameri R, Brust E, Suter M, Menz G (1994) Diagnostic value of recombinant *Aspergillus fumigatus* allergen I/a for skin testing and serology. J Allergy Clin Immunol 93:1–11

Niederberger V, Horak F, Vrtala S, Spitzauer S, Krauth MT, Valent P, Reisinger J, Pelzmann M, Hayek B, Kronqvist V, Gafvelin G, Gronlund H, Purohit A, Suck R, Fiebig H, Cromwell O, Pauli G, van Hage-Hamsten M, Valenta R (2004) Vaccination with genetically engineered allergens prevents progression of allergic disease. Proc Natl Acad Sci USA 101(Suppl 2):14677–14682

Niederberger V, Niggemann B, Kraft D, Spitzauer S, Valenta R (2002) Evolution of IgM, IgE and IgG(1-4)antibody responses in early childhood monitored with recombinant allergen components: implications for class switch mechanisms. Eur J Immunol 32:576–584

Niederberger V, Ring J, Rakoski J, Jager S, Spitzauer S, Valent P, Horak F, Kundi M, Valenta R (2007) Antigens drive memory IgE responses in human allergy via the nasal mucosa. Int Arch Allergy Immunol 142:133–144

Niemi M, Jylhä S, Laukkanen ML, Söderlund H, Mäkinen-Kijunen S, Kallio JM, Hakulinen N, Haahtela T, Takkinen K, Rouvinen J (2007) Molecular interactions between a recombinant IgE antibody and the beta-lactoglobulin allergen. Structure 15:1413–1421

Niespodziana K, Focke-Tejkl M, Linhart B, Civaj V, Blatt K, Valent P, van Hage M, Grönlund H, Valenta R (2011) A hypoallergenic cat vaccine based on Fel d 1-derived peptides fused to hepatitis B PreS. J Allergy Clin Immunol [Epub ahead of print]

Noon L (1911) Prophylactic inoculation against hay fever. Lancet 1:1572–1573

Norman PS, Ohman JL Jr, Long AA, Creticos PS, Gefter MA, Shaked Z, Wood RA, Eggleston PA, Hafner KB, Rao P, Lichtenstein LM, Jones NH, Nicodemus CF (1996) Treatment of cat allergy with T-cell reactive peptides. Am J Respir Crit Care Med 154:1623–1628

Padavattan S, Flicker S, Schirmer T, Madritsch C, Randow S, Reese G, Vieths S, Lupinek C, Ebner C, Valenta R, Markovic-Housley Z (2009) J Immunol 1822141–1822151

Paronchi P, Macchia D, Piccini MP, Biswas P, Simonelli C, Maggi E, Ricci M, Ansari AA, Romagnani S (1991) Allergen- and bacterial amtigen-specific T-cell clones established from atopic donors show a different profile of cytokine production. Proc Natl Acad Sci USA 15:4538–4542

Pauli G, Larsen TH, Rak S, Horak F, Pastorello E, Valenta R, Purohit A, Arvidsson M, Kavina A, Schroeder JW, Mothes N, Spitzauer S, Montagut A, Galvain S, Melac M, André C, Poulsen LK, Malling HJ (2008) Efficacy of recombinant birch pollen vaccine for the treatment of birch-allergic rhinoconjunctivitis. J Allergy Clin Immunol 122(5):951–960

Peters SP, Ferguson G, Deniz Y, Reisner C (2006) Uncontrolled asthma: a review of the prevalence, disease burden and options for treatment. Respir Med 100:1139–1151

Platts-Mills TA (2005) Asthma severity and prevalence: an ongoing interaction between exposure, hygiene, and lifestyle. PLoS Med 2:e34

Prausnitz C, Kuestner J (1921) Studien über die Überempfindlichkeit. Centralbe F Bakt 1 ABT Orig 86:160–168

Purohit A, Niederberger V, Kronqvist M, Horak F, Gronneberg R, Suck R, Weber B, Fiebig H, van Hage M, Pauli G, Valenta R, Cromwell O (2008) Clinical effects of immunotherapy with genetically modified recombinant birch pollen Bet v 1 derivatives. Clin Exp Allergy 38:1514–1525

Radulovic S, Calderon MA, Wilson D, Durham S (2010) Sublingual immunotherapy for allergic rhinitis. Cochrane Database Syst Rev 12:CD002893

Rak S (2009) Clinical results with a hypoallergenic recombinant birch pollen allergen derivative. Presented at 27th Congr, EAACI 2009, Warsaw, June 6–10

Raz E, Tighe H, Sato Y, Corr M, Dudler JA, Roman M, Swain SL, Spiegelberg HL, Carson DA (1996) Preferential induction of a Th1 immune response and inhibition of specific IgE antibody formation by plasmid DNA immunization. Proc Natl Acad Sci USA 93:5141–5145

Rocklin RE, Sheffer AL, Greineder DK, Melmon KL (1980) Generation of antigen-specific suppressor cells during allergy desensitization. N Engl J Med 302:1213–1219

Scadding GK, Brostoff J (1986) Low dose sublingual therapy in patients with allergic rhinitis due to house dust mite. Clin Allergy 16:483–491

Schmitz N, Dietmeier K, Bauer M, Maudrich M, Utzinger S, Muntwiler S (2009) Displaying Fel d1 on virus-like particles prevents reactogenicity despite greatly enhanced immunogenicity: a novel therapy for cat allergy. J Exp Med 206:1941–1955

Schumann A, Fiedler M, Dahmen U, Grosse-Wilde H, Roggendorf, M, Lindemann M (2007) Cellular and humoral immune response to a third generation hepatitis B vaccine. J Viral Hepat 14:592–598

Secrist H, Chelen CJ, Wen Y, Marshall JD, Umetsu DT (1993) Allergen immunotherapy decreases interleukin 4 production in CD + T cells from allergic individuals. J Exp Med 1:2123–2130

Sehon LZ, Mohapatra SS (1992) Induction of IgE antibodies in mice with recombinant grass pollen antigens. Immunology 76:158–163

Simons FE, Shikishima Y, Van Nest G, Eiden JJ, HayGlass KT (2004) Selective immune redirection in humans with ragweed allergy by injecting Amb a 1 linked to immunostimulatory DNA. J Allergy Clin Immunol 113:1144–1151

Siskind GW, Paul WE, Benacerraf B (1966) Studies on the effect of the carrier molecule on antihapten antibody synthesis. I. Effect of carrier on the nature of the antibody synthesized. J Exp Med 123:673–688

Stull A, Cooke RA, Tenant J (1933) The allergen content of protein extracts: Its determination and deterioration. J Allergy 4:455

Touart MD (1922) Hay fever; Desensitization by ingestion of pollen protein. NY Med J 116:199

Twaroch TE, Focke M, Civaj V, Weber M, Balic N, Mari A, Ferrara R, Quirce S, Spitzauer S, Swoboda I, Valenta R (2011) Carrier-bound, non-allergenic Ole e 1 peptides for vaccination against olive pollen allergy. J Allergy Clin Immunol [Epub ahead of print]

Urbanek R, Burgelin KH, Kahle S, Kuhn W, Wahn U (1990) Oral immunotherapy with grass pollen in enterosoluble capsules. A prospective study of the clinical and immunological response. Eur J Pediatr 149:545–550

Valenta R (2002) The future of antigen-specific immunotherapy of allergy. Nat Rev Immunol 2:446–453

Valenta R, Duchene M, Vrtala S, Birkner T, Ebner C, Hirschwehr R, Breitenbach M, Rumpold H, Scheiner O, Kraft D (1991) Recombinant allergens for immunoblot diagnosis of tree-pollen allergy. J Allergy Clin Immunol 88:889–894

Valenta R, Ball T, Focke M, Linhart M, Mothes N, Niederberger V, Spitzauer S, Swoboda I, Vrtala S, Westritsching K, Kraft D (2004) Immunotherapy of allergic disease. Adv Immunol 82:105–153

Valenta R, Ferreira F, Focke-Tejkl M, Linhart B, Niederberger V, Swoboda I, Vrtala S (2010) From allergen genes to allergy vaccines. Annu Rev Immunol 28:211–241

Valenta R, Niespodziana K, Focke-Tejkl M, Marth K, Huber H, Neubauer A, Niederberger V (2011) Recombinant allergens: what does the future hold? J Allergy Clin Immunol 127(4):860–864

van Neerven RJ, Knol EF, Ejrnaes A, Wurtzen PA (2006) IgE-mediated allergen presentation and blocking antibodies: regulation of T-cell activation in allergy. Int Arch Allergy Immunol 141:119–129

Vercelli D (2006) Mechanisms of the hygiene hypothesis–molecular and otherwise. Curr Opin Immunol 18:733–737

Walker JW, Adkinson J (1917) Studies on staphylococcus *pyogens aureus*, albus and citreus and on *Micrococcus tetragenous* and *M. catarrhalis*. J Med Res 35:391

Wide L, Bennich H, Johansson SG (1967) Diagnosis of allergy by an in vitro test for allergen antibodies. Lancet 2:1105–1107

Wyman M (1872) Autumnal Catarrh. Hurd and Houghton, Cambridge

Yunginger JW, Gleich GJ (1973) Seasonal changes in serum and nasal IgE concentrations. J Allergy Clin Immunol 51:174–186

Zoss AR, Koch CA, RS Hirose (1937) Alum-ragweed precipitate: preperation and clinical investigation; preliminary report. J Allergy 8:329–335

Passive Immunization with Allergen-Specific Antibodies

Sabine Flicker, Elisabeth Gadermaier, Christoph Madritsch and Rudolf Valenta

Abstract The induction of allergen-specific IgG antibodies has been identified as a major mechanism responsible for the reduction of allergic inflammation in allergic patients treated by allergen-specific immunotherapy. Several studies suggest that allergen-specific IgG antibodies induced by vaccination with allergens block mast cell and basophil degranulation, IgE-facilitated allergen presentation to T cells and IgE production. The availability of recombinant allergens and technologies for the production of recombinant human antibodies allows engineering of allergen-specific antibodies which can be used for passive immunization (i.e., therapy) and eventually for the prevention of allergy (i.e., prophylaxis). This chapter summarizes data supporting the possible use of allergen-specific antibodies for treatment and prophylaxis. Finally, concrete approaches for the treatment and prevention of allergy based on blocking antibodies are envisioned.

Abbreviations

SIT	Specific immunotherapy
APC	Antigen presenting cell
FcεRI	High-affinity IgE receptor
scFv	Single-chain antibody fragment
Fab	Antibody fragment
FcγR	IgG Fc receptor
FcRn	Neonatal Fc receptor
BAL	Broncho alveolar lavage
AHR	Airway hyper-responsiveness

S. Flicker (✉) · E. Gadermaier · C. Madritsch · R. Valenta
Division of Immunopathology, Department of Pathophysiology and Allergy Research, Center for Pathophysiology, Infectiology and Immunology, Vienna General Hospital, Medical University of Vienna, Waehringer Guertel 18-20, 1090 Vienna, Austria
e-mail: sabine.flicker@meduniwien.ac.at

Current Topics in Microbiology and Immunology (2011) 352: 141–159
DOI: 10.1007/82_2011_143

Published Online: 18 June 2011

OVA	Ovalbumin
i.v.	Intravenous
i.p.	Intraperitoneal
s.c.	Subcutaneous
SPR	Surface plasmon resonance
ADCC	Antibody dependent cell-mediated cytotoxicity

Contents

1 Background

The usefulness of IgG antibodies for passive immunization was demonstrated for the first time nearly 120 years ago. Passive immunization was applied to treat different infectious diseases, e.g., rabies, diphtheria and tetanus (von Behring and Kitasato 1991) (Sawyer 2000). Using the technology of passive serum transfer developed by Prausnitz and Kuestner (1921) for investigating mechanisms of allergic inflammation, Cooke et al. discovered that allergen-specific IgG antibodies that were induced by specific immunotherapy (SIT) were able to inhibit immediate inflammatory responses. In fact, they could demonstrate that allergen-specific IgG antibodies which block allergen-induced immediate allergic inflammation were transferable by simple serum injections from a treated to an untreated patient (Cooke 1935).

Even before it became technically possible to produce large amounts of defined allergen-specific IgG antibodies, a few studies provided evidence for the feasibility of using allergen-specific IgG antibodies for passive immunization. It was demonstrated for immunotherapy with ragweed extract that higher allergen doses were tolerated by patients who received combined passive and active immunotherapy (Bernstein et al. 1979). In order to prevent side effects, bee venom-allergic patients were pre-treated with beekeeper gammaglobulin to accept higher doses of venom (Muller et al. 1986; Bousquet et al. 1987).

The analysis of mechanisms underlying SIT with natural allergen extracts has been facilitated by the availability of recombinant allergens and defined epitopes. Moreover, several immunotherapy studies have been conducted with purified recombinant allergens, allergen-derived peptides and genetically modified allergens allowing a better understanding of the importance of blocking antibodies for successful treatment (Valenta et al. 2010; Larche et al. 2006).

2 Beneficial Role of Allergen-Specific Blocking IgG Antibodies

Allergen-specific IgG antibodies may suppress allergic immune responses and allergic inflammation through at least three different modes of action which are summarized in Fig. 1. First, they can inhibit immediate allergic inflammation by competing with mast cell-bound IgE antibodies for allergen binding and thus inhibit effector cell degranulation. A beneficial effect (i.e., reduction of degranulation) may be also achieved by co-cross-linking of mast cell-bound IgE and IgG by allergens (Fig. 1a). Second, allergen-specific IgG antibodies can compete with IgE bound to antigen presenting cells (APC) and thus prevent IgE-facilitated allergen presentation to T cells and thus T cell activation (Fig. 1b). Finally, allergen-specific IgG may capture allergens before they can induce IgE production (Fig. 1c) (Flicker and Valenta 2003; Wachholz and Durham 2004; Larche et al. 2006).

Cross-linking of allergens by FcεRI-bound IgE on mast cells or basophils is a key event in allergic inflammation. During the last decades it has been repeatedly shown by several clinical studies that SIT-induced allergen-specific IgG antibodies suppress allergen-induced mast cell degranulation and thus immediate allergic inflammation (Cooke 1935; Loveless 1940; Niederberger et al. 2004; Jutel et al. 2005; Klimek et al. 2005; Pauli et al. 2008; Purohit et al. 2008). IgG antibodies induced by SIT with a particular allergen source or allergen may also cross-protect against cross-reactive allergens. In this context it has been found that immunotherapy with birch pollen extract also protects against allergy to hazel and alder pollen (Petersen et al. 1988). More recently, it has been demonstrated that IgG induced by SIT with recombinant hypoallergenic derivatives of the major birch pollen allergen Bet v 1 inhibited basophil degranulation by Bet v 1-related food allergens (Niederberger et al. 2007a). Interestingly, SIT-induced IgG antibodies do not need to recognize exactly the same epitopes as those which are recognized by IgE. In fact, it has been shown that also IgG induced against new epitopes can block IgE binding as long as these antibodies occupy parts of the IgE epitopes or cause steric inhibition of IgE binding (Pree et al. 2007; Gadermaier et al. 2010a). It should be also stated at this point that the ability of a "blocking antibody" to

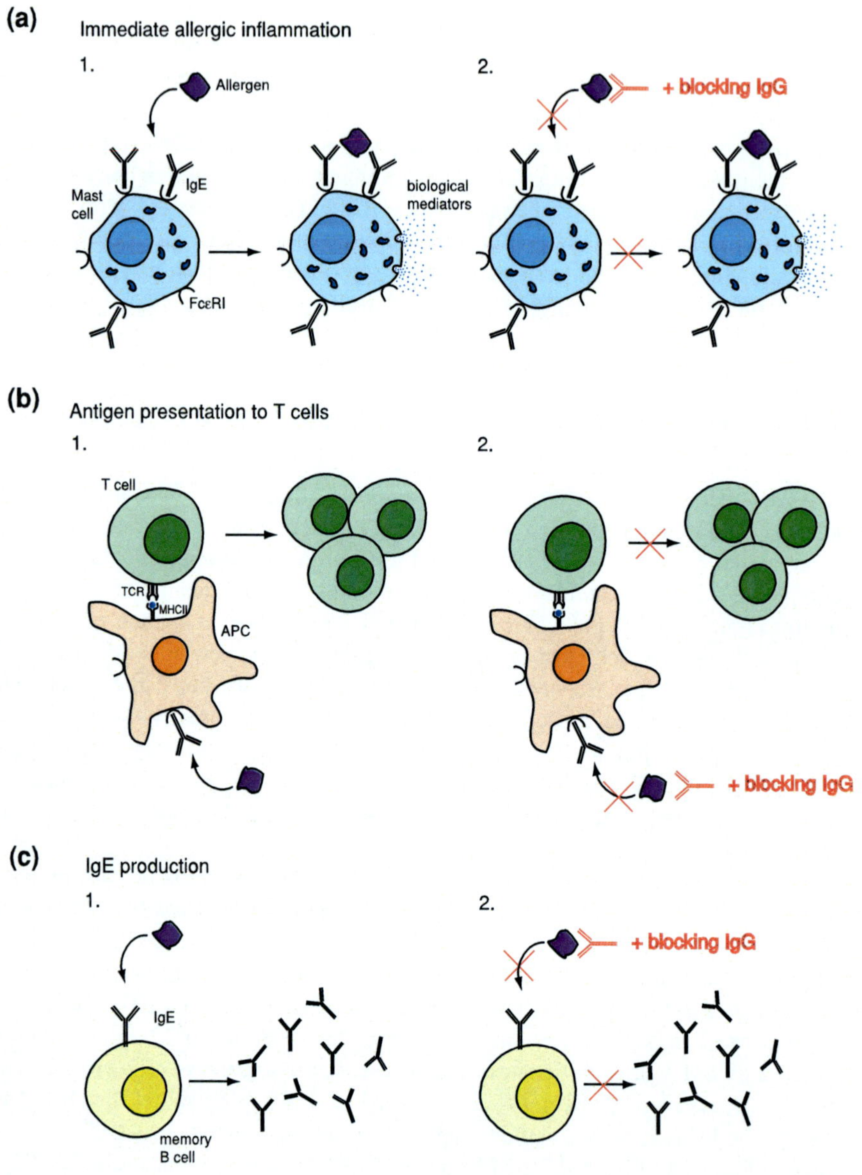

Fig. 1 *Summary of the beneficial roles of allergen-specific blocking IgG antibodies.* **a** Allergen-specific IgG captures allergen before it can cross-link mast cell-bound IgE and thus suppresses immediate allergic inflammation. **b** Allergen-specific IgG prevents allergens from being presented by IgE-facilitated antigen presentation to T cells and thus reduces T cell activation. **c** Allergen-specific IgG binds allergen and thus prevents allergens to activate IgE-producing cells

Table 1 Essential features for protective antibodies

Feature	References
Epitope specificity and titer	Flicker and Valenta (2003), Flicker et al. (2009)
Cross-reactivity	Valenta et al. (1996), Gieras et al. (2011)
Affinity	Jakobsen et al. (2004, 2005), Padavattan et al. (2009), Gieras et al. (2011)
Half-life and clearance	Akilesh et al. (2007), Jeffris (2009)
Binding to Fc receptors	Malbec and Daeron (2007)
Safety	Presta (2006), Hansel et al. (2010)

compete with IgE for allergen recognition does not at all depend on its isotype or subclass but only depends on its epitope specificity, affinity and titer. The latter statement is supported by defined mechanistic experiments performed with purified antibodies and allergens and cultured effector cells (Table 1). For example, defined human monoclonal allergen-specific IgG antibodies gained by hybridoma techniques or combinatorial library technology have been shown to inhibit IgE from binding to allergens and to suppress allergen-induced basophil degranulation (Visco et al. 1996; Flicker et al. 2002; Jylha et al. 2009; Padavattan et al. 2009). However, there is also evidence for another protective effect of allergen-specific IgG. It has been reported that concomitant binding of IgG and IgE antibodies to the same allergen may down-regulate effector cell responses through co-cross-linking of IgE and IgG receptors (Malbec and Daeron 2007; Mertsching et al. 2008). These studies have been performed mainly in murine models whereas for human immunotherapy studies no evidence for down-regulation of effector cell activation by co-cross-linking has been found so far (Ejrnaes et al. 2006).

Moreover, allergen-specific IgG antibodies are responsible for the reduction of IgE-facilitated antigen presentation by preventing the binding of allergen to APC-bound IgE antibodies resulting in decreased T cell activation. T cell activation is crucial for the development and perpetuation of the allergic immune response, and is also directly linked to the late-phase response as well as chronic inflammation of the airways (Larche et al. 2006).

In 1999, it was demonstrated that IgE-mediated allergen presentation to birch allergen-specific T cells was inhibited by IgG from sera of birch SIT patients, but not by IgG from patients who had received grass pollen-specific SIT, suggesting that an allergen-specific factor in their sera inhibited the IgE-mediated allergen presentation (van Neerven et al. 1999). The inhibitory effect was shown to be present in the IgG fraction of the birch SIT sera. This study and a follow-up study of sera from a placebo-controlled birch SIT study demonstrated that 100- to 1,000-fold higher allergen doses are needed to activate birch allergen-specific T cells after SIT (van Neerven et al. 2004). Confirmation came from another study demonstrating that blocking of allergen-IgE binding to B cells was mediated through IgG antibodies that were induced through grass pollen SIT and more recently by SIT with recombinant hypoallergenic Bet v 1 derivatives (Wachholz et al. 2003; Pree et al. 2010).

Thirdly, it has been shown that the induction of allergen-specific IgG antibodies by SIT is associated with a suppression of the boost of secondary IgE production by allergen contact. It is well-established that allergic patients exhibit strong increases of allergen-specific IgE levels after seasonal allergen exposure (Henderson et al. 1975; Niederberger et al. 2007b). A suppression of the rise of allergen-specific IgE during the pollen season in patients after SIT was noted in several studies (Mothes et al. 2003; Niederberger et al. 2004; Creticos et al. 2006). Since allergen-specific IgG decline relatively quickly after discontinuation of SIT it has been speculated that the suppression of IgE boosts by several courses of SIT administered for two or more years may be responsible for the long-term effect of SIT after its discontinuation (Gadermaier et al. 2011).

3 Isolation and Characterization of Allergen-Specific IgG Antibodies for Therapy and Prevention

The availability of recombinant purified major allergens of high clinical relevance provides a solid basis for the application of technologies for the isolation, characterization and production of allergen-specific therapeutic antibodies (Valenta and Kraft 1995, 2002). Phage display, combinatorial libraries and hybridoma techniques have enhanced our ability to obtain monoclonal recombinant antibodies (Huse et al. 1989; McCafferty et al. 1990; Winter et al. 1994).

One strategy to obtain "blocking antibodies or antibody derivatives" is to isolate IgE antibody fragments–scFvs or IgE Fabs– from allergic patients (Steinberger et al. 1996; Flicker et al. 2002; Jylha et al. 2009). Due to the lack of the constant region, these fragments cannot bind to the FcεRs and hence do not elicit IgE-mediated effects. Another strategy is to generate IgE antibody fragments and convert them into complete human IgG antibodies by engineering the IgE variable region onto an IgG constant region. These antibodies combine two important characteristics that may be relevant. They may block IgE binding to the allergen and in addition may bind to FcγRs thus mediating co-cross-linking and silencing of effector cells or allergen uptake and clearance.

One example for a conversion of an allergen-specific IgE Fab into an IgG_1 antibody is an IgE Fab specific for grass pollen allergen Phl p 2 obtained by combinatorial cloning from an allergic patient. This antibody inhibited patients' IgE binding to Phl p 2 and Phl p 2-induced histamine release from basophils of grass pollen allergic patients (Flicker et al. 2002; Padavattan et al. 2009). Nevertheless, it has been observed that single IgG antibodies that were derived from allergic patients IgE did not block polyclonal IgE binding to the allergen (Flicker et al. 2000, 2006).

Another possibility for obtaining allergen-specific monoclonal antibodies is conventional cell cloning technology. For example, monoclonal allergen-specific IgG antibodies have been isolated by EBV-transformation of allergen-specific B cells of a SIT-treated patient (Visco et al. 1996; Lebecque et al. 1997; Denepoux et al. 2000). However, as yet no human cell line producing allergen-specific IgE has been described.

Some essential features of allergen-specific IgG antibodies with protective potential are summarized in Table 1. The probably most important properties that make an IgG antibody a protective IgG antibody are epitope specificity and titer.

3.1 Epitope Specificity and Titer

It has been demonstrated that the blocking capacity of an allergen-specific antibody depends on its ability to occupy IgE binding sites or to bind in close vicinity so that there is steric hindrance of IgE binding (Flicker and Valenta 2003; Gieras et al. 2011).

In fact, SIT with allergen extracts can induce a large variety of IgG antibodies of which certain often do not even react with allergens, others recognize allergens but do not inhibit IgE binding and only some block IgE recognition (Flicker and Valenta 2003). Since SIT also induces "useless" IgG responses it has not been possible to associate the induction of IgG antibodies directly with clinical improvement (Djurup and Malling 1987; Birkner et al. 1990; Bodtger et al. 2005). Allergen-specific IgG antibodies which do not inhibit IgE binding to the allergen (Flicker et al. 2008) have been described and there is even evidence for IgG antibodies which may enhance IgE binding to allergens (Denepoux et al. 2000). Both reports clearly demonstrate that there are non-blocking IgG recognizing the wrong epitopes and it is not surprising that such antibodies have no therapeutic effect even when they are present in molar excess. The latter may also explain why certain allergic patients mount large amounts of allergen-specific IgG antibody responses but nevertheless suffer from allergy. Thus simple measurements of the allergen-specific IgG antibodies will not be sufficient surrogate markers for the clinical outcome of SIT.

However, if allergen-specific IgG antibodies have the correct epitope specificity and can inhibit IgE binding to the allergen, their protective effect will be greater if their concentration and titer is high.

It has been claimed that mainly allergen-specific IgG_4 antibodies are responsible for therapeutic effects during SIT (Aalberse et al. 1983). However, several studies demonstrate that the blocking activity of therapy-induced IgG antibodies does not reside exclusively in the IgG_4 fraction. Blocking antibodies of the IgG_1 subclass have been described (Visco et al. 1996; Flicker et al. 2002) and it has been shown that IgG_4-depleted sera retained their blocking activity (Ejrnaes et al. 2004).

Interestingly, it has turned out that the vast majority of allergens contain conformational IgE epitopes which are difficult to characterize because this requires sophisticated technologies e.g., three-dimensional structure analysis. With the application of structural biology methods first structures of complexes consisting of allergens and specific antibodies have been solved. The birch pollen allergen, Bet v 1, the bee venom allergen, Api m 2 (hyaluronidase) and the cockroach allergen Bla g 2, were co-crystallized with recombinant mouse IgG Fabs (Mirza et al. 2000; Padavattan et al. 2007; Li et al. 2008). Furthermore, the major bovine milk allergen, β-lactoglobulin and the major grass pollen allergen Phl p 2 were crystallized in complexes with recombinant human IgE Fabs (Niemi et al. 2007; Padavattan et al. 2009). These allergen-antibody complexes gave us for the first time insight in the molecular interaction between allergen and antibodies and revealed the nature of conformational IgE epitopes (Niemi et al. 2007; Padavattan et al. 2009).

3.2 *Cross-Reactivity*

Another important feature of an allergen-specific protective antibody is its cross-reactivity to homologous allergens present in related species. This finding is of great importance because IgE antibodies from allergic patients often displayed cross-reactivity to allergens from other allergen sources (Valenta et al. 1996; Radauer et al. 2008). So far, several monoclonal human and murine IgG blocking antibodies were demonstrated to cross-react with homologous allergens from related species (Visco et al. 1996; Lebecque et al. 1997; Flicker et al. 2002; Gieras et al. 2011) and were even shown to inhibit patients' IgE to related allergens (Gieras et al. 2011).

3.3 *Affinity*

Aside from epitope specificity, the affinity of antibodies for the given epitopes is an important factor. Affinity is perceived as the strength of binding and can be calculated from the quotient of dissociation rate and association rate. Moreover, the kinetics of an antibody/allergen complex is of great importance because the kinetics determines the on and off rates of formed complexes. Nowadays, the determination of the affinity and the kinetics of such complexes can be assessed by surface plasmon resonance (SPR) (Padavattan et al. 2009). When targeting protective antibodies applicable for passive immunotherapy high-affinity and low-dissociation rates are preferable. Determinations by SPR revealed that Bet v 1-specific IgG antibodies gained from allergic patients who had undergone immunotherapy had high affinities recorded in the nM range and hence reside in the same range as Bet v 1-specific IgE gained from the same patient (Jakobsen et al. 2004, 2005).

Recently, a human monoclonal IgG antibody specific for the major grass pollen allergen Phl p 2 has been engineered by grafting the variable domain of the corresponding IgE onto the human IgG_1 constant region. This antibody showed an extremely high affinity to Phl p 2 and strongly inhibited allergic patients IgE binding to the allergen as well as allergen-induced basophil degranulation (Padavattan et al. 2009). Murine antibodies recognizing peptides derived from the major IgE binding site of the major birch pollen allergen, Bet v 1 also showed high affinity to Bet v 1 (Gieras et al. 2011). Interestingly, these antibodies inhibited patients IgE binding but were less potent in inhibiting allergen-induced basophil degranulation.

The pairing of heavy and light chains also has an influence on the affinity and specificity of an antibody. Affinity of antibodies can be modified by pairing the original VH sequence with different VL sequences. Kim and Hong reported about an enhancement of affinity of a humanized monoclonal antibody after light chain shuffling (Kim and Hong 2007). For allergen-specific human IgE antibodies there is some evidence that the heavy chain determines allergen-specificity (Laffer et al. 2001; Rojas et al. 2004; Christensen et al. 2009; Gadermaier et al. 2010b). It is therefore quite possible, that the affinity of allergen-specific antibodies can be increased by shuffling of light chains.

3.4 Half-Life and Clearance

The affinity of a therapeutic allergen-specific antibody is not only important for the effective blocking of IgE but also affects other parameters. For example, high affinity of a therapeutic antibody would decrease dosing and frequency of administration, and thus reduce costs of treatment. Several reports describe different methods for improving affinity constants of antibodies toward their antigens. It could be shown that error-prone PCR using an excess of guanine and/or thymine resulted in the retrieval of antibody fragments with significantly improved binding affinities for the corresponding antigen (Persson et al. 2008). The same authors demonstrated in a former study that the change of several residues situated in the paratope of an antibody was critical for the strength of the binding affinity (Persson et al. 2006). Aside from the random mutagenesis strategy another method called "codon-based mutagenesis" has been described. The principle of this targeted approach is that specifically the CDRs are mutated (Glaser et al. 1992). Utilizing this technique Wu et al. succeeded in improving the affinity of an anti-angiogenic antibody by greater than 90-fold (Wu et al. 1998). It turned out that targeted mutagenesis in the CDR 3 led to the greatest affinity improvements due to the diminished off rate of the antibodies (Finlay et al. 2009).

Besides the efforts to improve the affinity constants of antibodies for the given antigen, many studies focus on understanding the factors that affect the pharmacokinectics of monoclonal antibodies, a field that is summarized by the term Fc engineering. The goal is the protection of monoclonal IgG antibodies from rapid clearance from the body, a prerequisite for effective passive immunization. Much effort has been made to prolong the survival of applied IgG including protection of antibody degradation through binding to Fc-receptors, e.g., neonatal Fc receptor (FcRn) and Fcγ receptors (FcγR). Several studies describe IgG stabilization by FcRn to their serum persistence by recycling internalized IgG to the cell surface (Ghetie et al. 1996; Akilesh et al. 2007; Roopenian and Akilesh 2007). In this context it turned out that human IgG_1, IgG_2 and IgG_4 per se exhibit longer elimination half-lives than IgG_3 a fact that is attributed to the binding differences to FcRn, as result of a single amino acid difference in the FcRn binding domain (Ghetie and Ward 2002). In accordance, attempts to alter the human IgG_1 antibody sequences, i.e., a single mutation in the CH2–CH3 region of the Fc part, led to affinity improvement of the human FcRn which was shown by Biacore analysis but also by in vivo studies in cynomogulus monkeys (Yeung et al. 2009). Nevertheless, the authors admitted that the increase of the affinity is not always associated with lower clearance (Yeung et al. 2009). Besides the cynomogulus monkey model which is well-known to be appropriate for investigating the half-lives of human IgG antibodies because the monkey FcRn binds human IgG, a human FcRn transgenic mouse model has been developed to evaluate the pre-clinical pharmacokinetics of human therapeutic antibodies (Petkova et al. 2006).

Another emerging issue is that the kind of glycosylation, e.g., galactose, fucose, N-acetylglucosamine has a strong impact on the half-life of the antibody (Jefferis 2009a). Different glycosylation patterns were easily achieved by using different expression systems (mammalian cells, yeasts, plants, insect cells and prokaryotes). The most widely used production cell lines for human therapeutic IgG antibodies are currently mammalian cells because the glycosylation pattern of assembled antibodies almost resembles the naturally glycosylated antibodies. Nevertheless, recombinant antibodies produced in well-established hamster or mouse cell lines like CHO, NSO and Sp2/0 usually have small quantities of unnatural glycoforms bearing the risk to be immunogenic and thus be cleared quicker by forming immune complexes (Jefferis 2009b). Therefore first efforts have been made to create genetically modified CHO cells or as alternative, yeast lines that use human enzymes for glycosylation to produce recombinant glycosylated human IgG antibodies with high-structural fidelity with the natural IgG antibodies (Jefferis 2009b).

The route of antibody application e.g., topical administration or systemic treatment is also discussed to influence the in vivo half-life of antibodies. It turned out that antibody titers in the BAL fluid of naïve BALB/C mice 48 h after intranasal instillation are hardly detectable whereas antibodies administered by i.v. route are maintained for several months in the sera (Sehra et al. 2003).

It is further reported that complete IgG antibodies in general are beneficial compared to antibody fragments like scFvs or Fabs due to their extended half-lives (Presta 2008). However, if neutralizing antibodies without eliciting any Fc-mediated effects are in favor antibody fragments became again of interest despite their short half-life. Several attempts have been made to prolong serum half-life of antibody fragments including linkage to polyethylene glycol (PEGylation) (Chapman et al. 1999; Constantinou et al. 2010) or linkage to albumin (Constantinou et al. 2010).

3.5 Binding to Fc Receptors

An interesting question is whether allergen-specific IgG antibodies besides simply competing for epitopes on allergens may exert their beneficial roles also via binding to FcγR.

In this context, it has been shown in OVA-sensitized mice that complete OVA-specific IgG2a and not OVA-specific F(ab)$_2$ suppressed inflammation indicating that FcγR-mediated mechanisms may be responsible for the repression (Sehra et al. 2003). FACS analysis clearly showed that alveolar macrophages are the main population responsible for the OVA capture by binding to IgG and FcγR on these cells. In parallel, a two-fold increase in INF-γ-secreting T cells was observed in IgG-treated mice (Sehra et al. 2003). However, it is also possible that complete antibodies were more efficient simply due to their longer half-life.

Strait et al. obtained results in a murine model suggesting that besides allergen interception by IgG antibodies (i.e., FcγR-mediated cellular uptake of allergen) also cross-linking of FcεRI to the inhibitory FcγRIIb through the allergen/IgG/IgE complex contributes to the inhibitory effect of administered IgG antibodies. They concluded that FcεRI/FcγRIIb cross-linking makes an important contribution when blocking IgG levels are limited but is redundant when blocking IgG antibody concentrations are high relative to concentrations of antigen in mice (Strait et al. 2006). Another recent report indicated that co-administration of mouse IgE and mouse IgG prevented mast cell degranulation in BALB/c mice whereas no IgG-dependent inhibition of mast cell degranulation was observed in FcγRIIB$^{-/-}$ mice (Uermosi et al. 2010).

For the human system, there is relatively little evidence that cross-linking of the FcεRI to the inhibitory IgG receptor FcγRIIb indeed plays a role in inhibiting histamine release. There are data from cultured human mast cells and basophils (Zhu et al. 2002; Tam et al. 2004; Zhang et al. 2004) and from in vivo studies using transgenic mice expressing human FcεRα (Allen et al. 2007). By investigating the inhibitory role of FcγRIIb of cat allergic patients who have received SIT, Cady et al. found evidence that FcγRIIA may be involved in the inhibition of basophil activation (Cady et al. 2010).

However, the investigation of the potential role of FcγR co-cross-linking in reducing allergen sensitivity in patients receiving immunotherapy failed to provide any evidence for this mechanism in allergic patients (Ejrnaes et al. 2006).

The choice of the isotype/subclass of a therapeutic allergen-specific antibody may be driven by several considerations. IgG$_1$ antibodies are often used as therapeutic antibodies. They have a long in vivo half-life but have been proven to be effective in activation of ADCC and complement activation (Jefferis 2007). Both are certainly not desired features although allergic patients develop allergen-specific IgG$_1$ in the course of SIT without showing signs of inflammation. Most likely, allergen-specific IgG$_4$ antibodies that just activate FcγRI and FcγRIIIa depending on the allotype of the receptor and/or the glycoform of the IgG$_4$ antibody but do not activate complement represent the most desirable subclass for passive immunization against allergens (Jefferis 2007, 2009b). In fact, allergen-specific IgG_4 is the prominent subclass associated with successful SIT, does not activate complement and can pass the placental barrier (Flicker et al. 2009) and thus may eventually protect children from becoming sensitized.

3.6 Safety of Recombinant Monoclonal Antibodies

Considerable efforts have been made in the last years to reduce side effects of therapeutic monoclonal antibodies. Among the side effects, immunogenicity is a major problem because it may lead to the development of antibodies against administered antibodies resulting in immune complexes, hypersensitivity or accelerated clearance of the applied antibodies. For decreasing immunogenicity of applied non-human antibodies different strategies like humanization, "resurfacing" (only surface-accessible framework amino acids are altered to human ones while the CDR and buried amino acids remain from parental rodent antibody) or SDR grafting (only a subset of CDR residues that are involved in binding of the antibody called "specificity-determining regions" is altered) have been suggested (Presta 2006). De-immunization, another technology, means the identification and alteration of potential T cell epitopes present in the antibody without reducing the binding affinity (Presta 2006). The availability of fully human monoclonal antibodies by phage display library or transgenic mice is another possibility to produce therapeutic antibodies with low immunogenicity. To date, just few examples of human therapeutic antibodies exist that have passed the safety requirements (FDA approval) and are already used in the field of oncology, psoriasis and asthma (Corren et al. 2010; Hansel et al. 2010). The lessons learned from the other fields may be translated to the field of type I allergy.

4 Proof of Concept Testing in Animal Models

In order to investigate the in vivo efficacy of passive administration of allergen-specific IgG antibodies a few murine models have been established so far. It has been shown that topical or systemic administration of allergen-specific IgG antibodies reduces allergic inflammation in sensitized mice (Sehra et al. 2003; Moerch et al. 2006; Strait et al. 2006) (Flicker unpublished data). Sera of OVA-sensitized mice that received anti-OVA specific IgG antibodies exhibited significantly reduced OVA-specific IgE levels, significantly reduced levels of leukocytes and eosinophil granulocytes in BALs and significantly reduced AHR to methacholine (Sehra et al. 2003; Moerch et al. 2006). The efficacy of a single administration of allergen-specific IgG antibodies was confirmed by data from mice sensitized to

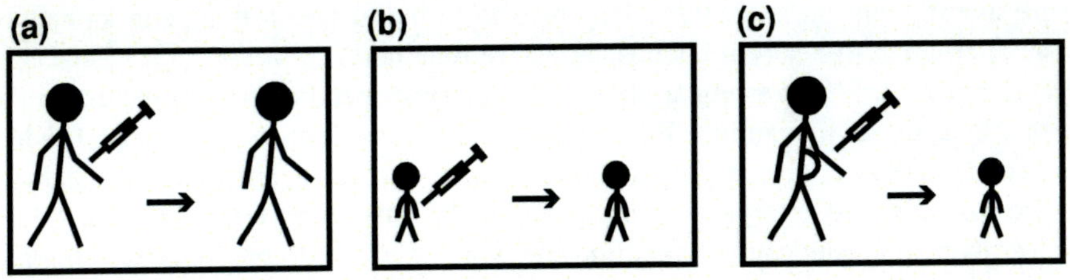

Fig. 2 *Envisaged therapeutic and prophylactic immunization with allergen-specific antibodies.* **a** Therapeutic application may protect allergic patients from symptoms in the course of allergen contact. **b** Prophylactic application shortly after birth to children may protect against allergic sensitization. **c** Application of allergen-specific IgG antibodies to pregnant mother may lead to diaplacental transfer to children and protect them against allergic sensitization after birth

three of the most important seasonal allergens, the major grass and birch pollen allergens, Phl p 1, Phl p 5 and Bet v 1 (Flicker unpublished data).

Very few data exist so far for prophylactic treatment with allergen-specific antibodies, i.e., administration of allergen-specific antibodies before sensitization to allergen takes place. It has already been demonstrated in experimental animal models and in clinical studies that prenatal induction of allergen-specific IgG antibodies protects against allergen-induced sensitization and allergic inflammation in the offspring (Glovsky et al. 1991; Jenmalm and Bjorksten 2000; Uthoff et al. 2003; Polte and Hansen 2008; Polte et al. 2008; Flicker et al. 2009; Victor et al. 2010).

It will thus be very interesting to explore if passive immunization of pregnant mothers or new born children with allergen-specific IgG antibodies can suppress allergic sensitization (Fig. 2).

5 Possible Application of Allergen-Specific IgG for Therapy and Prophylaxis

With the availability of defined reagents (i.e., clinically relevant allergens) and new technologies (e.g., combinatorial cloning technologies and large-scale production of fully human antibodies) it should be possible to produce allergen-specific human IgG antibodies for the clinically most relevant allergens. The following concrete applications for allergen-specific IgG antibodies can be envisaged. First, it should be possible to treat seasonal allergies by passive immunization of allergic patients shortly before the beginning of the pollen season (Fig. 2a). Since human allergen-specific IgG_4 antibodies have a half-life of approximately 21 days it is quite possible that allergic patients can be protected by a single passive immunization for a full pollen season. Perennial allergies are perhaps not easy to treat by passive immunization because repeated injections may be needed, but also Omalizumab, an injected therapeutic anti-IgE is successfully used to treat such patients (Holgate et al. 2009). It may thus well be envisioned that passive immunization against allergens which elicit severe asthma attacks may be an alternative to heavy immunosuppressive treatment.

Another very interesting application of allergen-specific IgG antibodies may be prophylactic immunization (Fig. 2). There is some evidence that prenatal induction of allergen-specific IgG antibodies may protect against allergen-induced sensitization and allergic inflammation in the offspring (Glovsky et al. 1991; Jenmalm and Bjorksten 2000; Flicker et al. 2009). For prophylaxis, allergen-specific IgG may be either administered to pregnant women who transmit the protective IgG via their placenta to the children (Fig. 2c) or directly to the children shortly after birth in order to prevent allergic sensitization (Fig. 2b).

References

Aalberse RC, van der Gaag R, van Leeuwen J (1983) Serologic aspects of IgG4 antibodies. I. Prolonged immunization results in an IgG4-restricted response. J Immunol 130(2):722–726

Akilesh S, Christianson GJ, Roopenian DC, Shaw AS (2007) Neonatal FcR expression in bone marrow-derived cells functions to protect serum IgG from catabolism. J Immunol 179(7): 4580–4588

Allen LC, Kepley CL, Saxon A, Zhang K (2007) Modifications to an Fcgamma-Fcvarepsilon fusion protein alter its effectiveness in the inhibition of FcvarepsilonRI-mediated functions. J Allergy Clin Immunol 120(2):462–468

Bernstein IL, Michael JG, Malkiel S, Sweet LC, Brackett RG (1979) Immunoregulatory function of specific IgG. II. Clinical evaluation of combined active and passive immunotherapy. Int Arch Allergy Appl Immunol 58(1):30–37

Birkner T, Rumpold H, Jarolim E, Ebner H, Breitenbach M, Skvaril F, Scheiner O, Kraft D (1990) Evaluation of immunotherapy-induced changes in specific IgE, IgG and IgG subclasses in birch pollen allergic patients by means of immunoblotting. Correlation with clinical response. Allergy 45(6):418–426

Bodtger U, Ejrnaes AM, Hummelshoj L, Jacobi HH, Poulsen LK, Svenson M (2005) Is immunotherapy-induced birch-pollen-specific IgG4 a marker for decreased allergen-specific sensitivity? Int Arch Allergy Immunol 136(4):340–346

Bousquet J, Fontez A, Aznar R, Robinet-Levy M, Michel FB (1987) Combination of passive and active immunization in honeybee venom immunotherapy. J Allergy Clin Immunol 79(6):947–954

Cady CT, Powell MS, Harbeck RJ, Giclas PC, Murphy JR, Katial RK, Weber RW, Hogarth PM, Johnson S, Bonvini E, Koenig S, Cambier JC (2010) IgG antibodies produced during subcutaneous allergen immunotherapy mediate inhibition of basophil activation via a mechanism involving both FcgammaRIIA and FcgammaRIIB. Immunol Lett 130(1–2):57–65

Chapman AP, Antoniw P, Spitali M, West S, Stephens S, King DJ (1999) Therapeutic antibody fragments with prolonged in vivo half-lives. Nat Biotechnol 17(8):780–783

Christensen PA, Danielczyk A, Ravn P, Larsen M, Stahn R, Karsten U, Goletz S (2009) Modifying antibody specificity by chain shuffling of V/V between antibodies with related specificities. Scand J Immunol 69(1):1–10

Constantinou A, Chen C, Deonarain MP (2010) Modulating the pharmacokinetics of therapeutic antibodies. Biotechnol Lett 32(5):609–622

Cooke R (1935) Serological evidence of immunity with coexisting sensitization in hay fever type of humanallergy. J Exp Med 62:733–750

Corren J, Busse W, Meltzer EO, Mansfield L, Bensch G, Fahrenholz J, Wenzel SE, Chon Y, Dunn M, Weng HH, Lin SL (2010) A randomized, controlled, phase 2 study of AMG 317, an IL-4Ralpha antagonist, in patients with asthma. Am J Respir Crit Care Med 181(8):788–796

Creticos PS, Schroeder JT, Hamilton RG, Balcer-Whaley SL, Khattignavong AP, Lindblad R, Li H, Coffman R, Seyfert V, Eiden JJ, Broide D (2006) Immunotherapy with a ragweed-toll-like receptor 9 agonist vaccine for allergic rhinitis. N Engl J Med 355(14):1445–1455

Denepoux S, Eibensteiner PB, Steinberger P, Vrtala S, Visco V, Weyer A, Kraft D, Banchereau J, Valenta R, Lebecque S (2000) Molecular characterization of human IgG monoclonal antibodies specific for the major birch pollen allergen Bet v 1. Anti-allergen IgG can enhance the anaphylactic reaction. FEBS Lett 465(1):39–46

Djurup R, Malling HJ (1987) High IgG4 antibody level is associated with failure of immunotherapy with inhalant allergens. Clin Allergy 17(5):459–468

Ejrnaes AM, Bodtger U, Larsen JN, Svenson M (2004) The blocking activity of birch pollen-specific immunotherapy-induced IgG4 is not qualitatively superior to that of other IgG subclasses. Mol Immunol 41(5):471–478

Ejrnaes AM, Svenson M, Lund G, Larsen JN, Jacobi H (2006) Inhibition of rBet v 1-induced basophil histamine release with specific immunotherapy -induced serum immunoglobulin G: no evidence that FcgammaRIIB signalling is important. Clin Exp Allergy 36(3):273–282

Finlay WJ, Cunningham O, Lambert MA, Darmanin-Sheehan A, Liu X, Fennell BJ, Mahon CM, Cummins E, Wade JM, O'Sullivan CM, Tan XY, Piche N, Pittman DD, Paulsen J, Tchistiakova L, Kodangattil S, Gill D, Hufton SE (2009) Affinity maturation of a humanized rat antibody for anti-RAGE therapy: comprehensive mutagenesis reveals a high level of mutational plasticity both inside and outside the complementarity-determining regions. J Mol Biol 388(3):541–558

Flicker S, Valenta R (2003) Renaissance of the blocking antibody concept in type I allergy. Int Arch Allergy Immunol 132(1):13–24

Flicker S, Vrtala S, Steinberger P, Vangelista L, Bufe A, Petersen A, Ghannadan M, Sperr WR, Valent P, Norderhaug L, Bohle B, Stockinger H, Suphioglu C, Ong EK, Kraft D, Valenta R (2000) A human monoclonal IgE antibody defines a highly allergenic fragment of the major timothy grass pollen allergen, Phl p 5: molecular, immunological, and structural characterization of the epitope-containing domain. J Immunol 165(7):3849–3859

Flicker S, Steinberger P, Norderhaug L, Sperr WR, Majlesi Y, Valent P, Kraft D, Valenta R (2002) Conversion of grass pollen allergen-specific human IgE into a protective IgG(1) antibody. Eur J Immunol 32(8):2156–2162

Flicker S, Steinberger P, Ball T, Krauth MT, Verdino P, Valent P, Almo S, Valenta R (2006) Spatial clustering of the IgE epitopes on the major timothy grass pollen allergen Phl p 1: importance for allergenic activity. J Allergy Clin Immunol 117(6):1336–1343

Flicker S, Steinberger P, Eibensteiner PB, Lebecque S, Kraft D, Valenta R (2008) Molecular characterization of a human immunoglobulin G4 antibody specific for the major birch pollen allergen, Bet v 1. Clin Exp Allergy 38 (2):365–373

Flicker S, Marth K, Kofler H, Valenta R (2009) Placental transfer of allergen-specific IgG but not IgE from a specific immunotherapy-treated mother. J Allergy Clin Immunol 124(6):1358–1360 e1

Gadermaier E, Flicker S, Aberer W, Egger C, Reider N, Focke M, Vrtala S, Kundi M, Valenta R (2010a) Analysis of the antibody responses induced by subcutaneous injection immunotherapy with birch and Fagales pollen extracts adsorbed onto aluminum hydroxide. Int Arch Allergy Immunol 151(1):17–27

Gadermaier E, Flicker S, Steinberger P, Valenta R (2010b) Evidence that the heavy-chain determines the specificity of IgE antibodies in allergy. 14th international congress of immunology, Kansai, Japan, International Immunology Meeting Abstracts (2010) 22 (Suppl 1 Pt 1): i138–i141. doi:10.1093/intimm/dxq108

Gadermaier E, Staikuniene J, Scheiblhofer S, Thalhamer J, Kundi M, Westritschnig K, Swoboda I, Flicker S, Valenta R (2011) Recombinant allergen-based monitoring of antibody responses during injection grass pollen immunotherapy and after 5 years of discontinuation. Allergy doi:10.1111/j.1398-9995.2011.02592.x

Ghetie V, Ward ES (2002) Transcytosis and catabolism of antibody. Immunol Res 25(2):97–113

Ghetie V, Hubbard JG, Kim JK, Tsen MF, Lee Y, Ward ES (1996) Abnormally short serum half-lives of IgG in beta 2-microglobulin-deficient mice. Eur J Immunol 26(3):690–696

Gieras A, Cejka P, Blatt K, Focke-Tejkl M, Linhart B, Flicker S, Stoecklinger A, Marth K, Drescher A, Thalhamer J, Valent P, Majdic O, Valenta R (2011) Mapping of conformational IgE epitopes with peptide-specific monoclonal antibodies reveals simultaneous binding of different IgE antibodies to a surface patch on the major birch pollen allergen, Bet v 1. J Immunol 186(9):5333–5344

Glaser SM, Yelton DE, Huse WD (1992) Antibody engineering by codon-based mutagenesis in a filamentous phage vector system. J Immunol 149(12):3903–3913

Glovsky MM, Ghekiere L, Rejzek E (1991) Effect of maternal immunotherapy on immediate skin test reactivity, specific rye I IgG and IgE antibody, and total IgE of the children. Ann Allergy 67(1):21–24

Hansel TT, Kropshofer H, Singer T, Mitchell JA, George AJ (2010) The safety and side effects of monoclonal antibodies. Nat Rev Drug Discov 9(4):325–338

Henderson LL, Larson JB, Gleich GJ (1975) Maximal rise in IgE antibody following ragweed pollination season. J Allergy Clin Immunol 55(1):10–15

Holgate S, Smith N, Massanari M, Jimenez P (2009) Effects of omalizumab on markers of inflammation in patients with allergic asthma. Allergy 64(12):1728–1736

Huse WD, Sastry L, Iverson SA, Kang AS, Alting-Mees M, Burton DR, Benkovic SJ, Lerner RA (1989) Generation of a large combinatorial library of the immunoglobulin repertoire in phage lambda. Science 246(4935):1275–1281

Jakobsen CG, Bodtger U, Kristensen P, Poulsen LK, Roggen EL (2004) Isolation of high-affinity human IgE and IgG antibodies recognising Bet v 1 and Humicola lanuginosa lipase from combinatorial phage libraries. Mol Immunol 41(10):941–953

Jakobsen CG, Bodtger U, Poulsen LK, Roggen EL (2005) Vaccination for birch pollen allergy: comparison of the affinities of specific immunoglobulins E, G1 and G4 measured by surface plasmon resonance. Clin Exp Allergy 35(2):193–198

Jefferis R (2007) Antibody therapeutics: isotype and glycoform selection. Expert Opin Biol Ther 7(9):1401–1413

Jefferis R (2009a) Glycosylation as a strategy to improve antibody-based therapeutics. Nat Rev Drug Discov 8(3):226–234

Jefferis R (2009b) Recombinant antibody therapeutics: the impact of glycosylation on mechanisms of action. Trends Pharmacol Sci 30(7):356–362

Jenmalm MC, Bjorksten B (2000) Cord blood levels of immunoglobulin G subclass antibodies to food and inhalant allergens in relation to maternal atopy and the development of atopic disease during the first 8 years of life. Clin Exp Allergy 30(1):34–40

Jutel M, Jaeger L, Suck R, Meyer H, Fiebig H, Cromwell O (2005) Allergen-specific immunotherapy with recombinant grass pollen allergens. J Allergy Clin Immunol 116(3): 608–613

Jylha S, Makinen-Kiljunen S, Haahtela T, Soderlund H, Takkinen K, Laukkanen ML (2009) Selection of recombinant IgE antibodies binding the beta-lactoglobulin allergen in a conformation-dependent manner. J Immunol Methods 350(1–2):63–70

Kim SJ, Hong HJ (2007) Guided selection of human antibody light chains against TAG-72 using a phage display chain shuffling approach. J Microbiol 45(6):572–577

Klimek L, Bachert C, Doemer C, Meyer H, Narkus A (2005) Specific immunotherapy with recombinant brich pollen allergen rBet v 1-FV is clinically efficacious. Allergy Clin Immunol Int (suppl 1):15

Laffer S, Steinberger P, Kraft D, Valenta R (2001) Promiscuous use of light chains by human IgE antibodies specific for three major grass pollen allergens. Int Arch Allergy Immunol 124(1–3): 29–30

Larche M, Akdis CA, Valenta R (2006) Immunological mechanisms of allergen-specific immunotherapy. Nat Rev Immunol 6(10):761–771

Lebecque S, Dolecek C, Laffer S, Visco V, Denepoux S, Pin JJ, Guret C, Boltz-Nitulescu G, Weyer A, Valenta R (1997) Immunologic characterization of monoclonal antibodies that modulate human IgE binding to the major birch pollen allergen Bet v 1. J Allergy Clin Immunol 99(3):374–384

Li M, Gustchina A, Alexandratos J, Wlodawer A, Wunschmann S, Kepley CL, Chapman MD, Pomes A (2008) Crystal structure of a dimerized cockroach allergen Bla g 2 complexed with a monoclonal antibody. J Biol Chem 283(33):22806–22814

Loveless M (1940) Immunological studies of pollinosis. I. The presence of two antibodies related to the same pollen antigen in the serum of treated hay fever patients. J Immunol 38:25–50

Malbec O, Daeron M (2007) The mast cell IgG receptors and their roles in tissue inflammation. Immunol Rev 217:206–221

McCafferty J, Griffiths AD, Winter G, Chiswell DJ (1990) Phage antibodies: filamentous phage displaying antibody variable domains. Nature 348(6301):552–554

Mertsching E, Bafetti L, Hess H, Perper S, Giza K, Allen LC, Negrou E, Hathaway K, Hopp J, Chung J, Perret D, Shields M, Saxon A, Kehry MR (2008) A mouse Fcgamma-Fcepsilon protein that inhibits mast cells through activation of FcgammaRIIB, SH2 domain-containing inositol phosphatase 1, and SH2 domain-containing protein tyrosine phosphatases. J Allergy Clin Immunol 121(2):441–447

Mirza O, Henriksen A, Ipsen H, Larsen JN, Wissenbach M, Spangfort MD, Gajhede M (2000) Dominant epitopes and allergic cross-reactivity: complex formation between a Fab fragment of a monoclonal murine IgG antibody and the major allergen from birch pollen Bet v 1. J Immunol 165(1):331–338

Moerch U, Haahr Hansen M, Vest Hansen NJ, Rasmussen LK, Oleksiewicz MB, Frandsen TP, Haurum JS, Bregenholt S (2006) Allergen-specific polyclonal antibodies reduce allergic disease in a mouse model of allergic asthma. Int Arch Allergy Immunol 140(3):261–269

Mothes N, Heinzkill M, Drachenberg KJ, Sperr WR, Krauth MT, Majlesi Y, Semper H, Valent P, Niederberger V, Kraft D, Valenta R (2003) Allergen-specific immunotherapy with a monophosphoryl lipid A-adjuvanted vaccine: reduced seasonally boosted immunoglobulin E production and inhibition of basophil histamine release by therapy-induced blocking antibodies. Clin Exp Allergy 33(9):1198–1208

Muller UR, Morris T, Bischof M, Friedli H, Skarvil F (1986) Combined active and passive immunotherapy in honeybee-sting allergy. J Allergy Clin Immunol 78(1 Pt 1):115–122

Niederberger V, Horak F, Vrtala S, Spitzauer S, Krauth MT, Valent P, Reisinger J, Pelzmann M, Hayek B, Kronqvist M, Gafvelin G, Gronlund H, Purohit A, Suck R, Fiebig H, Cromwell O, Pauli G, van Hage-Hamsten M, Valenta R (2004) Vaccination with genetically engineered allergens prevents progression of allergic disease. Proc Natl Acad Sci USA 101(suppl 2):14677–14682

Niederberger V, Reisinger J, Valent P, Krauth MT, Pauli G, van Hage M, Cromwell O, Horak F, Valenta R (2007a) Vaccination with genetically modified birch pollen allergens: immune and clinical effects on oral allergy syndrome. J Allergy Clin Immunol 119(4):1013–1016

Niederberger V, Ring J, Rakoski J, Jager S, Spitzauer S, Valent P, Horak F, Kundi M, Valenta R (2007b) Antigens drive memory IgE responses in human allergy via the nasal mucosa. Int Arch Allergy Immunol 142(2):133–144

Niemi M, Jylha S, Laukkanen ML, Soderlund H, Makinen-Kiljunen S, Kallio JM, Hakulinen N, Haahtela T, Takkinen K, Rouvinen J (2007) Molecular interactions between a recombinant IgE antibody and the beta-lactoglobulin allergen. Structure 15(11):1413–1421

Padavattan S, Schirmer T, Schmidt M, Akdis C, Valenta R, Mittermann I, Soldatova L, Slater J, Mueller U, Markovic-Housley Z (2007) Identification of a B-cell epitope of hyaluronidase, a major bee venom allergen, from its crystal structure in complex with a specific Fab. J Mol Biol 368(3):742–752

Padavattan S, Flicker S, Schirmer T, Madritsch C, Randow S, Reese G, Vieths S, Lupinek C, Ebner C, Valenta R, Markovic-Housley Z (2009) High-affinity IgE recognition of a conformational epitope of the major respiratory allergen Phl p 2 as revealed by X-ray crystallography. J Immunol 182(4):2141–2151

Pauli G, Larsen TH, Rak S, Horak F, Pastorello E, Valenta R, Purohit A, Arvidsson M, Kavina A, Schroeder JW, Mothes N, Spitzauer S, Montagut A, Galvain S, Melac M, Andre C, Poulsen

LK, Malling HJ (2008) Efficacy of recombinant birch pollen vaccine for the treatment of birch-allergic rhinoconjunctivitis. J Allergy Clin Immunol 122(5):951–960

Persson H, Lantto J, Ohlin M (2006) A focused antibody library for improved hapten recognition. J Mol Biol 357(2):607–620

Persson H, Wallmark H, Ljungars A, Hallborn J, Ohlin M (2008) In vitro evolution of an antibody fragment population to find high-affinity hapten binders. Protein Eng Des Sel 21(8):485–493

Petersen BN, Janniche H, Munch EP, Wihl JA, Bowadt H, Ipsen H, Lowenstein H (1988) Immunotherapy with partially purified and standardized tree pollen extracts. I. Clinical results from a three-year double-blind study of patients treated with pollen extracts either of birch or combinations of alder, birch and hazel. Allergy 43(5):353–362

Petkova SB, Akilesh S, Sproule TJ, Christianson GJ, Al Khabbaz H, Brown AC, Presta LG, Meng YG, Roopenian DC (2006) Enhanced half-life of genetically engineered human IgG1 antibodies in a humanized FcRn mouse model: potential application in humorally mediated autoimmune disease. Int Immunol 18(12):1759–1769

Polte T, Hansen G (2008) Maternal tolerance achieved during pregnancy is transferred to the offspring via breast milk and persistently protects the offspring from allergic asthma. Clin Exp Allergy 38(12):1950–1958

Polte T, Hennig C, Hansen G (2008) Allergy prevention starts before conception: maternofetal transfer of tolerance protects against the development of asthma. J Allergy Clin Immunol 122(5):1022–1030 e5

Prausnitz C, Küstner H (1921) Studien über die Überempfindlichkeit. Zbl Bakt 86:160–169

Pree I, Reisinger J, Focke M, Vrtala S, Pauli G, van Hage M, Cromwell O, Gadermaier E, Egger C, Reider N, Horak F, Valenta R, Niederberger V (2007) Analysis of epitope-specific immune responses induced by vaccination with structurally folded and unfolded recombinant Bet v 1 allergen derivatives in man. J Immunol 179(8):5309–5316

Pree I, Shamji MH, Kimber I, Valenta R, Durham SR, Niederberger V (2010) Inhibition of CD23-dependent facilitated allergen binding to B cells following vaccination with genetically modified hypoallergenic Bet v 1 molecules. Clin Exp Allergy 40(9):1346–1352

Presta LG (2006) Engineering of therapeutic antibodies to minimize immunogenicity and optimize function. Adv Drug Deliv Rev 58(5–6):640–656

Presta LG (2008) Molecular engineering and design of therapeutic antibodies. Curr Opin Immunol 20(4):460–470

Purohit A, Niederberger V, Kronqvist M, Horak F, Gronneberg R, Suck R, Weber B, Fiebig H, van Hage M, Pauli G, Valenta R, Cromwell O (2008) Clinical effects of immunotherapy with genetically modified recombinant birch pollen Bet v 1 derivatives. Clin Exp Allergy 38(9):1514–1525

Radauer C, Bublin M, Wagner S, Mari A, Breiteneder H (2008) Allergens are distributed into few protein families and possess a restricted number of biochemical functions. J Allergy Clin Immunol 121(4):847–852 e7

Rojas G, Talavera A, Munoz Y, Rengifo E, Krengel U, Angstrom J, Gavilondo J, Moreno E (2004) Light-chain shuffling results in successful phage display selection of functional prokaryotic-expressed antibody fragments to N-glycolyl GM3 ganglioside. J Immunol Methods 293(1–2):71–83

Roopenian DC, Akilesh S (2007) FcRn: the neonatal Fc receptor comes of age. Nat Rev Immunol 7(9):715–725

Sawyer LA (2000) Antibodies for the prevention and treatment of viral diseases. Antiviral Res 47(2):57–77

Sehra S, Pynaert G, Tournoy K, Haegeman A, Matthys P, Tagawa Y, Pauwels R, Grooten J (2003) Airway IgG counteracts specific and bystander allergen-triggered pulmonary inflammation by a mechanism dependent on Fc gamma R and IFN-gamma. J Immunol 171(4):2080–2089

Steinberger P, Kraft D, Valenta R (1996) Construction of a combinatorial IgE library from an allergic patient. Isolation and characterization of human IgE Fabs with specificity for the major timothy grass pollen allergen, Phl p 5. J Biol Chem 271(18):10967–10972

Strait RT, Morris SC, Finkelman FD (2006) IgG-blocking antibodies inhibit IgE-mediated anaphylaxis in vivo through both antigen interception and Fc gamma RIIb cross-linking. J Clin Invest 116(3):833–841

Tam SW, Demissie S, Thomas D, Daeron M (2004) A bispecific antibody against human IgE and human FcgammaRII that inhibits antigen-induced histamine release by human mast cells and basophils. Allergy 59(7):772–780

Uermosi C, Beerli RR, Bauer M, Manolova V, Dietmeier K, Buser RB, Kundig TM, Saudan P, Bachmann MF (2010) Mechanisms of allergen-specific desensitization. J Allergy Clin Immunol 126(2):375–383

Uthoff H, Spenner A, Reckelkamm W, Ahrens B, Wolk G, Hackler R, Hardung F, Schaefer J, Scheffold A, Renz H, Herz U (2003) Critical role of preconceptional immunization for protective and nonpathological specific immunity in murine neonates. J Immunol 171(7):3485–3492

Valenta R, Kraft D (1995) Recombinant allergens for diagnosis and therapy of allergic diseases. Curr Opin Immunol 7(6):751–756

Valenta R, Kraft D (2002) From allergen structure to new forms of allergen-specific immunotherapy. Curr Opin Immunol 14(6):718–727

Valenta R, Steinberger P, Duchene M, Kraft D (1996) Immunological and structural similarities among allergens: prerequisite for a specific and component-based therapy of allergy. Immunol Cell Biol 74(2):187–194

Valenta R, Ferreira F, Focke-Tejkl M, Linhart B, Niederberger V, Swoboda I, Vrtala S (2010) From allergen genes to allergy vaccines. Ann Rev Immunol 28:211–214

van Neerven RJ, Wikborg T, Lund G, Jacobsen B, Brinch-Nielsen A, Arnved J, Ipsen H (1999) Blocking antibodies induced by specific allergy vaccination prevent the activation of CD4 + T cells by inhibiting serum-IgE-facilitated allergen presentation. J Immunol 163(5):2944–2952

van Neerven RJ, Arvidsson M, Ipsen H, Sparholt SH, Rak S, Wurtzen PA (2004) A double-blind, placebo-controlled birch allergy vaccination study: inhibition of CD23-mediated serum-immunoglobulin E-facilitated allergen presentation. Clin Exp Allergy 34(3):420–428

Victor JR, Muniz BP, Fusaro AE, de Brito CA, Taniguchi EF, Duarte AJ, Sato MN (2010) Maternal immunization with ovalbumin prevents neonatal allergy development and up-regulates inhibitory receptor Fc gamma RIIB expression on B cells. BMC Immunol 11:11

Visco V, Dolecek C, Denepoux S, Le Mao J, Guret C, Rousset F, Guinnepain MT, Kraft D, Valenta R, Weyer A, Banchereau J, Labecque S (1996) Human IgG monoclonal antibodies that modulate the binding of specific IgE to birch pollen Bet v 1. J Immunol 157(2):956–962

von Behring E, Kitasato S (1991) The mechanism of diphtheria immunity and tetanus immunity in animals. 1890. Mol Immunol 28(12):1317 1319–1320

Wachholz PA, Durham SR (2004) Mechanisms of immunotherapy: IgG revisited. Curr Opin Allergy Clin Immunol 4(4):313–318

Wachholz PA, Soni NK, Till SJ, Durham SR (2003) Inhibition of allergen-IgE binding to B cells by IgG antibodies after grass pollen immunotherapy. J Allergy Clin Immunol 112(5):915–922

Winter G, Griffiths AD, Hawkins RE, Hoogenboom HR (1994) Making antibodies by phage display technology. Annu Rev Immunol 12:433–455

Wu H, Beuerlein G, Nie Y, Smith H, Lee BA, Hensler M, Huse WD, Watkins JD (1998) Stepwise in vitro affinity maturation of Vitaxin, an alphav beta3-specific humanized mAb. Proc Natl Acad Sci USA 95(11):6037–6042

Yeung YA, Leabman MK, Marvin JS, Qiu J, Adams CW, Lien S, Starovasnik MA, Lowman HB (2009) Engineering human IgG1 affinity to human neonatal Fc receptor: impact of affinity improvement on pharmacokinetics in primates. J Immunol 182(12):7663–7671

Zhang K, Kepley CL, Terada T, Zhu D, Perez H, Saxon A (2004) Inhibition of allergen-specific IgE reactivity by a human Ig Fcgamma-Fcepsilon bifunctional fusion protein. J Allergy Clin Immunol 114(2):321–327

Zhu D, Kepley CL, Zhang M, Zhang K, Saxon A (2002) A novel human immunoglobulin Fc gamma Fc epsilon bifunctional fusion protein inhibits Fc epsilon RI-mediated degranulation. Nat Med 8(5):518–521

Cell-Based Therapy in Allergy

Ulrike Baranyi, Martina Gattringer, Rudolf Valenta and Thomas Wekerle

Abstract IgE-mediated allergy is an immunological disorder occurring in response to otherwise harmless environmental antigens (i.e., allergens). Development of effective therapeutic or preventive approaches inducing robust tolerance toward allergens remains an unmet goal. Several experimental tolerance approaches have been described. The therapeutic use of regulatory T cells (Tregs) and the establishment of molecular chimerism are two cell-based strategies that are of particular interest. Treg therapy is close to clinical application, but its efficacy remains to be fully defined. Recent proof-of-concept studies demonstrated that transplantation of syngeneic hematopoietic stem cells modified in vitro to express a major allergen leads to molecular chimerism and robust allergen-specific tolerance. Here we review cell-based tolerance strategies in allergy, discussing their potentials and limitations.

Contents

U. Baranyi · M. Gattringer · T. Wekerle (✉)
Division of Transplantation, Department of Surgery, Vienna General Hospital, Medical University of Vienna, Vienna, Austria
e-mail: Thomas.Wekerle@meduniwien.ac.at

R. Valenta
Division of Immunopathology, Department of Pathophysiology, Center of Physiology and Pathophysiology, Medical University of Vienna, Vienna, Austria

Current Topics in Microbiology and Immunology (2011) 352: 161–179

DOI: 10.1007/82_2011_127

Published Online: 20 May 2011

1 Introduction

IgE-mediated allergic disorders are immunological hypersensitivity reactions. Allergic immune responses occur against environmental, otherwise innocuous antigens, known as allergens. Genetic and environmental factors influence susceptibility to allergic hypersensitivity (Akdis 2006; Vercelli 2008).

The only causative treatment available so far is allergen-specific immunotherapy (SIT), a vaccination strategy (Valenta 2002). Increasing doses of allergens (mostly in the form of crude extracts) are administered to allergic individuals with the goal to induce "desensitization". In this context, immunological tolerance in allergy was suggested to be defined as persistence of efficacy after treatment (Akdis and Akdis 2009). Numerous mechanisms have been suggested to show how SIT alters B cell and T cell responses. Mechanisms may vary depending on treatment protocol, route of administration and allergen preparation (Larche et al. 2006). SIT induces de novo humoral responses dominated by the production of protective allergen-specific IgG antibodies, mainly IgG4 (Nouri-Aria et al. 2004; Wachholz and Durham 2003). A Th2 to Th1 shift and induction of Tregs also contribute to effectiveness (Bohle 2008). SIT is, however, associated with limited effectiveness and considerable risks, as exemplified by anaphylactic reactions or therapy-induced sensitization to additional allergens when crude extracts are used (Valenta 2002). In addition to the need for more effective allergen-specific therapeutic strategies, prevention of allergy by prophylactic induction of tolerance is a major unmet need (Hamelmann et al. 2007).

Several experimental tolerance strategies have been described, with cell-based approaches having gained particular attention in recent years. This review discusses induction of tolerance through cell therapies as a possible approach to prevent and treat allergy.

2 Prevention of Allergy by Induction of Peripheral Tolerance

Peripheral, i.e., extrathymic, T cell tolerance is a critical mechanism of self-tolerance and can either occur by peripheral clonal deletion (Webb et al. 1990), anergy (Fathman and Lineberry 2007) or suppression (Sakaguchi 2005).

Potent tolerance models relying on peripheral tolerance have been developed. Conceptually, they suffer, however, from the drawback to have no mechanism in place to tolerize newly developing T cells and thus their effects are usually limited in duration (Wekerle et al. 2003).

2.1 Induction of Tolerance via the Mucosal Route

Specific non-responsiveness to inhaled and ingested allergens is a major goal in IgE-mediated allergy. Mucosal tolerance is induced through administration of antigens via the oral or nasal route (Faria and Weiner 2005). This phenomenon was reported very early as protection of systemic anaphylaxis was observed upon injection of hen's egg protein in guinea pigs having been fed with the antigen (Wells 1911). Two primary mechanisms of mucosal tolerance have been described. Low-dose antigen- feeding induces active suppression by generation of Tregs, high-dose feeding regimens induce anergy (Friedman and Weiner 1994). TGFß (transforming growth factor beta)-producing T helper type 3 (Th3) cells are a Treg subtype specifically induced upon antigen-feeding (reviewed in Faria and Weiner 2005). Beside T cell-mediated immunoregulation, induction of allergen-specific IgA antibodies is a prominent mechanism of oral tolerance (Challacombe and Tomasi 1980).

Mucosal tolerance via the respiratory tract is more relevant to inhalant allergens. High-dose intranasal exposure of one single dominant T cell epitope of the house dust mite allergen Der p 1 was sufficient to induce T cell anergy toward the whole Der p 1 allergen by linked suppression, a phenomenon prominently described in transplantation (Hoyne et al. 1993, 1999; Qin et al. 1993). Dominant T cell epitopes of different allergens and in different combinations have been investigated for intranasal application, resulting in reduction of allergen-specific IgE and IgG responses. However, allergen-specific isotypes are not completely eliminated and only short-term follow up was reported in these models (Hufnagl et al. 2005, 2008; Marazuela et al. 2008; Wild et al. 2007). Involvement of Tregs and a Th2 to Th1 shift are important mechanisms in these protocols (Hufnagl et al. 2008; Marazuela et al. 2008; Winkler et al. 2006).

2.2 Induction of Tolerance by Intradermal Peptide Application

Systemic subcutaneous administration of T cell peptides of the major cat allergen Fel d 1 (without adjuvant) successfully led to peripheral T cell tolerance in experimental models. Translation to the clinical setting employing intradermal administration of T cell peptides of Fel d 1, however, induced late asthmatic reactions in some patients (Briner et al. 1993; Haselden et al. 1999; Oldfield et al. 2002). T cell responses were diminished, but humoral responses toward the full length allergen persisted (Briner et al. 1993). In a novel transgenic mouse model of asthma mimicking the human situation systemic intradermal application of one Fel d 1 immunodominant peptide in pre-sensitized mice resulted in resolution of airway pathology through linked suppression, possibly through generation of Tregs (Campbell et al. 2009). To allow full assessment of the potential of T cell peptides as therapeutic vaccines, several parameters still need to be determined, such as optimum length and dose of peptides (Larche and Wraith 2005).

2.3 Tregs as Cell-Based Therapy in Allergy

Regulatory T cells play a critical role in maintaining self-tolerance (Sakaguchi and Powrie 2007). Numerous, incompletely defined, subpopulations of Tregs have been described, with CD4+CD25+FoxP3+ natural Tregs arising from the thymus, and adaptive/induced Tregs generated in the periphery playing major roles (Feuerer et al. 2009). Tregs regulate T cell and B cell responses and also innate immunity. Whether memory T cells are amenable to regulation by Tregs remains controversial (Levings et al. 2001; Yang et al. 2007). The therapeutic exploitation of Tregs has attracted enormous interest in recent years, fueled by hopes of developing antigen-specific treatments for transplant recipients, autoimmune diseases and allergies (Akl et al. 2008; Hutchinson et al. 2008; Riley et al. 2009). So far, however, the physiology of Tregs remains incompletely understood and their therapeutic potential largely unexplored (Schiopu and Wood 2008).

Several lines of evidence reveal a prominent role of Tregs in regulating, or preventing, respectively allergic immune responses. A role for T regulatory type 1 (Tr1) cells in modulating allergic immune responses has been found by comparing immune responses upon allergen exposure between healthy individuals and allergic patients (Akdis et al. 2004). Natural high exposure of venom allergen (phospholipase A2) induces a switch of specific Th1 and Th2 cells to Tr1 cells (Meiler et al. 2008). Tr1 cells are of special therapeutic interest, as they are currently under clinical investigation in bone marrow (BM) transplant recipients, as are natural Tregs (nTregs) (reviewed in Roncarolo and Battaglia 2007; Roncarolo et al. 2006; Schiopu and Wood 2008; Riley et al. 2009). First clinical trials using freshly isolated or expanded donor nTregs show encouraging results in the prevention of lethal graft versus host disease (GVHD) (Trzonkowski et al. 2009; Brunstein et al. 2011; Di Ianni et al. 2011) nTregs express the transcription factor forkhead box P3 (FoxP3) (Miyara et al. 2009) and play an indispensable role in maintaining self-tolerance (Sakaguchi et al. 2008). FoxP3-deficient patients suffering from immunodysregulation, polyendocrinopathy and enteropathy X-linked syndrome (IPEX) are affected by atopic disease, resulting in increased serum IgE levels, eosinophilia, eczema-like skin lesions and enhanced Th2 responses. This provides clear evidence that Fox P3-expressing Tregs play an essential role in suppression of Th2-driven immune responses in humans (Chatila 2005).

In experimental models in allergy, the therapeutic application of nTregs abolished allergic airway inflammation (Kearley et al. 2005, 2008; Leech et al. 2007). Transfer of nTregs resulted in reduction of allergen-specific IgE and a boost of IgG1 immunomodulation after nasal administration of Der p 1 in an IL-10 independent manner (Leech et al. 2007). In another model, ova-specific CD4+CD25+ T cells suppressed T cell responses in the lung but IgE responses were not altered in a preventive approach (Kearley et al. 2005). Features of chronic allergen-induced inflammation were resolved but established remodeling in the lung was not reversed and humoral responses to allergen were not altered (Kearley et al. 2008). Thus, the use of natural Tregs has a suppressive effect on allergic airway inflammation, but seems to be less effective in preventing IgE responses. Application of FoxP3-transduced polyclonal CD4+ cells is effective in models of autoimmunity and allo-transplantation (Chai et al. 2005; Jaeckel et al. 2005; Pilat et al. 2010). Using polyclonal transduced Tregs together with the application of a recombinant grass pollen allergen in preventive and therapeutic murine models, we observed that allergen-specific IgE was not significantly reduced and T cell responses were not suppressed (Baranyi, Pilat, Wekerle et al., unpublished data).

In summary, Treg therapy is of considerable interest for treating allergic diseases. Numerous basic biological questions still need to be resolved in this new field of investigation. Only then can the clinical potential of Treg therapy be adequately assessed.

3 Tolerance Induction by Hematopoietic Stem Cell Transplantation (HSCT)

Self-tolerance is mediated mostly by various subpopulations of hematopoietic cells (von Boehmer and Kisielow 2006). Chimerism-based tolerance strategies emulate this fundamental characteristic of physiologic self-tolerance with the aim of inducing tolerance toward introduced, disease-causing antigens (Fehr and Sykes 2008; Wekerle and Sykes 2001). Such chimerism protocols are the only strategies to reliably establish central tolerance, i.e., the intrathymic clonal deletion of antigen-specific thymocytes. Thereby they provide mechanisms not only for tolerizing pre-existing mature T cells through peripheral mechanisms (Bigenzahn et al. 2005; Wekerle et al. 2002), but also for continuously tolerizing the newly developing T cells constantly arising in the thymus (Wekerle et al. 1998; Wekerle and Sykes 2001). Moreover, chimerism is capable of inducing T cell, B cell and NK cell tolerance (Sykes et al. 1998), and also tolerance in pre-sensitized recipients (Colson et al. 2000). Tolerance induced by chimerism is thus of particular robustness and durability.

Two types of hematopoietic chimerism can be distinguished: cellular and molecular, with mixed chimerism being the most commonly used subtype of cellular chimerism. Allogeneic donor BM (containing HSC) is transplanted to establish mixed chimerism. In the case of molecular chimerism autologous (i.e., syngeneic in the rodent setting) HSC are transplanted after genetic modification ex vivo to express the disease-causing antigen(s) (Bagley et al. 2002a).

Advanced experimental protocols of cellular hematopoietic chimerism have been systematically developed for several decades. Translation to large animal models and the clinical setting have been accomplished for transplantation tolerance (Fehr and Sykes 2008). Thus, chimerism-based tolerance is conceptually and empirically an attractive tolerance strategy with demonstrated clinical potential.

3.1 Mixed Chimerism

Following transplantation of donor BM into appropriately conditioned recipients, donor and recipient hematopoiesis co-exists (>1 < 100% donor cells), leading to donor-specific tolerance (reviewed in Sykes 2001; Wekerle and Sykes 2001).

Subsequent to the early observation of chimerism as a natural phenomenon in cattle, the concept has been translated to numerous experimental models (Billingham et al. 1953; Owen 1945). At first myeloablative recipient conditioning was used (Ildstad and Sachs 1984), which has been extensively modified so that substantially milder regimens have since become available (Pree et al. 2007). Mixed chimerism was found to be preferable over full chimerism as it reduces the risk of graft versus host disease (GVHD) and is associated with superior immunocompetence (Singer et al. 1981; Sykes et al. 1988). The use of co-stimulation blockers (mostly CTLA4Ig and anti-CD40L) as part of BM transplantation (BMT) protocols allowed chimerism and tolerance to be induced with the mildest, least toxic conditioning protocols developed to date (Durham et al. 2000; Pree and Wekerle 2006; Snanoudj et al. 2006; Wekerle et al. 2000). Permanent engraftment of conventional BM doses without recipient irradiation, remained however, an important goal. Either unrealistic mega doses of BM (Blaha et al. 2005; Durham et al. 2000; Wekerle et al. 2000), or recipient myelosuppression (by irradiation or cytotoxic drugs) have been necessary (Adams et al. 2001; Blaha et al. 2003; Koporc et al. 2008; Takeuchi et al. 2004). Co-transplantation of recipient Tregs allowed for the first time the engraftment of conventional doses of fully allogeneic BM without any myelosuppressive recipient conditioning (Pilat et al. 2010; Pilat and Wekerle 2010).

The clinical potential of the mixed chimerism strategy has recently been emphasized by two pilot trials. In the first series, patients suffering from chronic renal insufficiency plus concomitant myeloma were simultaneously grafted with a kidney and with BM from an HLA-identical sibling (Bühler et al. 2002; Fudaba et al. 2006). Patients accepted the renal grafts without maintenance immunosuppression. In a subsequent trial, HLA-mismatched BM plus a kidney were transplanted into recipients with chronic renal failure (without concomitant malignancy) (Kawai et al. 2008; LoCascio et al. 2010). Four out of five patients became tolerant, with long-term preserved kidney graft function (reported follow up of up to 5 years; one patient lost his graft due to humeral rejection). These results provide clinical proof-of-concept that transplantation tolerance can be achieved through mixed chimerism (Pilat et al. 2009). Widespread application of this regimen is, however, prevented by the extensive myelosuppressive host conditioning which is required to allow even transient engraftment of HLA-mismatched BM and which is associated with substantial risks and toxicities. Therefore, more advanced, milder protocols that already exist in the rodent setting need to be translated to clinical use for routine application of the mixed chimerism strategy to become realistic.

3.2 Molecular Chimerism

Transplantation of syngeneic HSC that have been genetically modified in vitro to express disease-causing antigen(s) back into the same individual induces tolerance toward the introduced antigen(s). This gene therapy has been successfully employed in experimental models of allo- or xeno-transplantation and some selected autoimmune diseases. Autologous HSCT has the advantage compared to allogeneic HSCT that the risk of GVHD is avoided (Copelan 2006), and that the lower immunological barrier would allow milder host conditioning (Bagley and Iacomini 2003).

The safety issues associated with gene therapy, however, are a major drawback of molecular chimerism. Retro- or lentiviral vectors currently used for gene introduction into HSC cause substantial toxicity due to immune reactions or oncogenesis (Baum et al. 2003; Hacein-Bey-Abina et al. 2008). Recently, progress toward safer gene delivery has been reported (Aiuti et al. 2009; Mitsuyasu et al. 2009) and it is anticipated that acceptably safe vector systems will become available some time in the future.

3.2.1 Introduction of Allo- and Xeno- Genes to Establish Tolerance

Major histocompatibility complex (MHC) molecules are the primary target of immune responses in allotransplantation (Davidson and Diamond 2001; LeGuern 2007). Expression of single donor MHC class I and class II antigens can be sufficient for inducing tolerance toward fully allogeneic donors under certain circumstances, due to linked suppression and “infectious tolerance” (Frasca et al. 1997; Qin et al. 1993). Besides, certain alleles of MHC class I and II are strongly associated with the risk of developing autoimmune disease.

Donor MHC class I or class II genes transduced into recipient cells in vitro and transferred into recipients led to prolonged cardiac allografts survival (Madsen et al. 1988). Similarly, swine MHC class II DRB was integrated by retroviral transfer into murine and swine BM cells (BMC) in vitro (Emery et al. 1993; Shafer et al. 1991). By translating this method to a porcine in vivo model, prolonged renal allograft survival was achieved by transducing a single allogeneic MHC class II gene into recipient BMC (Emery et al. 1997; Sonntag et al. 2001).

In contrast, MHC class I gene transfer seems to be more difficult due to poor peptide presentation of MHC class I peptides (LeGuern 2007). The congeneic mouse strains B10.AKM (H-2K^k)-B10.MBR (H-2K^b)—differing in only one H-2K allele—serve as a model of allogeneic molecular chimerism. Several studies introducing the MHC class I (K^b) into murine BMC (K^k) showed hyporesponsiveness and prolongation of skin allografts (K^b). In these protocols low transduction efficiency at first resulted only in prolongation of skin grafts but not durable tolerance (Bagley et al. 2000; Fraser et al. 1995; Mayfield et al. 1997). By improving transduction efficiency of BMC by a different retroviral gene transfer system, stable multilineage molecular chimerism and long-term skin graft tolerance was achieved (Bagley et al. 2002b). Mechanistically, central thymic deletion plus peripheral mechanisms, including regulation by CD4+CD25+ Tregs, were shown to play a role in this model (Forman et al. 2005, 2006; Kang and Iacomini 2002) and existence of molecular blood chimerism is required for durable tolerance (Tian et al. 2006).

In xenotransplantation (pig to human), natural xenoantibodies against the carbohydrate epitope Gal α-1, 3-Gal (αgal) are an additional barrier. Thus both B cell and T cell tolerance are required for long-lasting acceptance of xenografts. Humans, Old World monkeys and Apes possess a diminished function of α1, 3-galactosyltransferase (αGT), the enzyme producing αgal (Galili et al. 1988). The αGT knockout mouse (GT^0) model (having IgG and IgM antibodies toward αgal) is used to study natural antibodies in xenotransplantation. By introduction of αGT into syngeneic BMC B cell tolerance through molecular chimerism can be studied. Long-term molecular chimerism and B cell tolerance were achieved even when mice were pre-sensitized with pig cells and cardiac grafts from αGT expressing mice were accepted in GT^0 mice (Bracy and Iacomini 2000, 2002; Bracy et al. 1998, 2001; Kearns-Jonker et al. 2004; Mitsuhashi et al. 2006). Autologous transduced BMC expressing αGT was also transplanted into rhesus monkeys and xenoantibody production was strongly reduced after sensitization with porcine cells (Fischer-Lougheed et al. 2006).

3.2.2 Introduction of Auto-Antigens to Establish Tolerance

Molecular chimerism has also been studied in selected autoimmune models (Alderuccio et al. 2003). In experimental autoimmune encephalomyelitis (EAE), a rodent model to study multiple sclerosis (Zamvil and Steinman 1990), genes encoding for myelin oligodendrocyte glycoprotein (MOG), phospholipid protein (PLP) , myelin basic protein (MBP) and antigens inducing EAE, were introduced into BMC and established tolerance in EAE (Chan et al. 2008; Xu and Scott 2004; Xu et al. 2006). In one study introduction of MBP resulted in worsening of the disease, possibly due to insufficient MBP expression (Peters et al. 2000). Introduction of one peptide epitope of MOG (MOG_{40-55}) fused to a murine MHC II-associated invariant chain into syngeneic BMC resulted in tolerance induction in preventive and therapeutic models reported recently (Eixarch et al. 2009).

In the NOD type I diabetes model autoreactive T cells respond to islet antigens (insulin, glutamic acid decarboxylase (GAD) and others). The MHC class II region in NOD mice encodes a single MHC class II molecule I-A^{g7} (homologue to human HLA-DQB1 lacking a charged amino acid at position 57 associated with susceptibility to develop type 1 diabetes) which confers susceptibility to spontaneous type I diabetes (Atkinson and Leiter 1999). Induction of molecular chimerism through transplantation of BM expressing a 'disease-resistant' MHC class II molecule prevented type I diabetes in NOD mice and was sufficient to restore normoglycemia after islet transplantation and led to central thymic deletion of autoreactive T cells (Tian et al. 2004a, 2007a).

3.3 Hematopoietic Stem Cell Transplantation and Allergy

Cases in which BM transplanted from allergic donors induced allergies in the recipient have been reported. In reverse, allergies have been described to be cured in allergic recipients receiving a BMT from a healthy donor, suggesting that BMT is an effective treatment for allergies (though of course not indicated for this disease). No systematic, prospective evaluation of these issues, however, is available (Hourinhane et al. 2005; Khan et al. 2009; Storek et al. 2011).

4 Induction of Tolerance via Molecular Chimerism in Allergy

Molecular chimerism is an effective strategy for tolerance toward allo- and autoantigens. We recently started to investigate this strategy for tolerance in allergy. As most clinically relevant allergens have been identified and are available as cDNAs (Valenta and Kraft 2002), and as only a limited number of allergens is relevant in any given patient (and even geographical) region, allergies seem particularly suited for the molecular chimerism approach.

4.1 Prevention of Allergy by Induction of Tolerance via Molecular Chimerism

In proof-of-concept studies, we developed a preventive experimental model for induction of tolerance via molecular chimerism (Baranyi et al. 2008). A clinically relevant grass pollen allergen, Phl p 5 (Vrtala et al. 1993), was employed as model allergen. Phl p 5 is highly immunogenic upon subcutaneous immunization with the adjuvant aluminiumhydroxide in wild type mice (BALB/c) (Linhart et al. 2007). For cell surface expression on HSC Phl p 5 was fused to a signal peptide and a transmembrane domain and ligated into a retroviral expression vector. Syngeneic BMC were transduced with recombinant retroviruses integrating Phl p 5 and thereafter Phl p 5-expressing BMC were transplanted into myeloablated syngeneic recipients. Mice transplanted with Phl p 5-transduced BM and mice of control groups were repeatedly immunized with recombinant (r) Phl p 5 and an unrelated allergen (rBet v 1) post BMT. BMT of Phl p 5-transduced cells resulted in stable long-term multilineage chimerism (follow-up approximately 9 months). Transduction of true HSC, already suggested by long-term multi-lineage chimerism, was confirmed through successful transplantation of BM taken from chimeras into secondary recipients (Down and Ploemacher 1993).

In this model durable tolerance was demonstrated by the complete absence of Phl p 5-specific IgE, IgA and IgG antibodies throughout follow up while high antibody responses to Bet v 1 were preserved. Tolerance at the effector cell levels in vitro and in vivo toward Phl p 5 was also achieved. T cell tolerance toward the introduced allergen was demonstrated by unresponsivess in proliferation assays. These results have been confirmed by transplanting BM transduced with a distinct, unrelated allergen (Bet v 1) (Gattringer, Wekerle et al., unpublished). Again lasting molecular chimerism and allergen-specific tolerance were observed. Therefore molecular chimerism is uniquely potent in establishing complete and permanent tolerance at the T cell, B cell and effector cell levels in experimental type I allergy (Baranyi et al. 2008, 2009).

4.2 Anticipated Impediments to Translate Molecular Chimerism to the Clinical Setting and Possible Solutions

Safety aspects have high priority in prophylactic approaches in allergy (Kulig et al. 1999). Therefore non-toxic protocols are a pre-requisite for translation. The experimental protocol employed in our proof-of-principle study entails several components that cannot be applied clinically, such as retroviral gene transfer, irradiation and others. We propose that solutions to these problems can be envisioned (Fig. 1).

4.2.1 Moving to Safer Protocols

Retro- or lentiviral vector-based delivery to integrate transgenes is efficient but associated with oncogenicity and mutagenesis (Thomas et al. 2003). The hyperactive *Sleeping Beauty* DNA transposon was shown to integrate transgenes in a robust and stable manner into CD34+ HSC reconstituted in mice and was even successful to modify T cells before transfer in humans in a gene therapy approach (VandenDriessche et al. 2009). Therefore DNA transposons are a potential safer alternative for integrating genes into HSC.

In constrast to murine models, in which chimerism needs to persist in order to maintain robust tolerance (Tian et al. 2006), transient mixed chimerism was

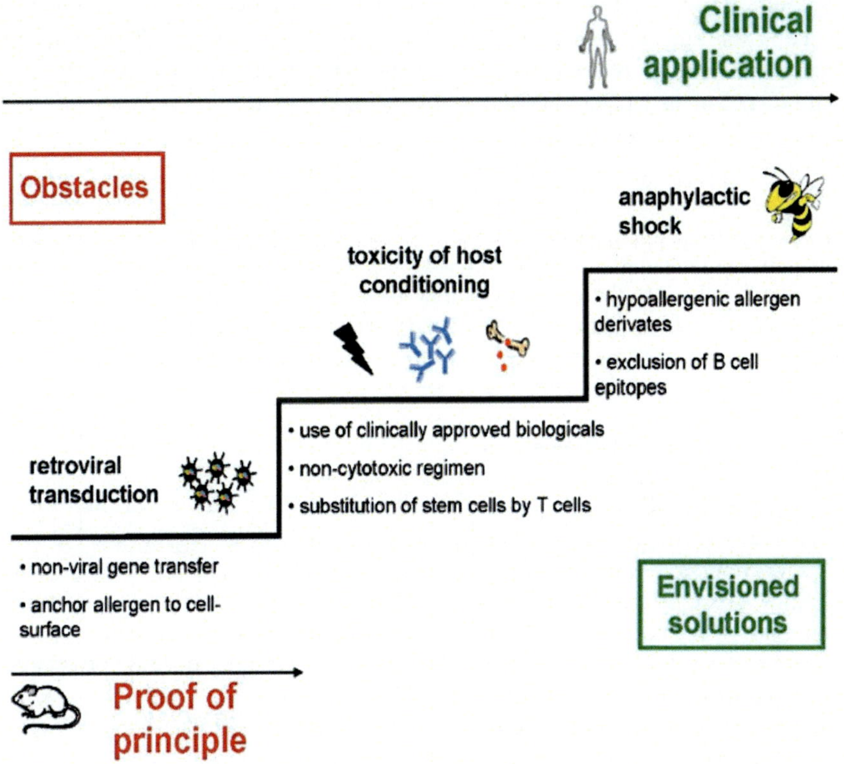

Fig. 1 Obstacles and envisioned solutions of cell based therapy by molecular chimerism, describing the hurdles on the way to clinical application starting with a proof-of-principle experiment in the mouse model

sufficient for tolerance in monkey models and clinical trials (Kawai et al. 2008; Ochiai et al. 2007). Thus, if transient chimerism suffices episomal, non-integrating delivery can be used, or antigens can be anchored directly to the cell surface (Belting and Wittrup 2009; Thomas et al. 2003; Yolcu et al. 2002).

In our proof-of-principle study, mice received a myeloablative dose of irradiation. Reduction of irradiation resulted in lower chimerism levels, but mice were still tolerant long-term (Baranyi, Wekerle et al., unpublished). In other models of molecular and mixed chimerism very mild experimental protocols have already been developed and could be translated to the allergy system in the future (Blaha et al. 2003; Eixarch et al. 2009; Forman et al. 2005; Tian et al. 2008; Wekerle et al. 2000; Pilat et al. 2010).

Application of the co-stimulation blocker anti-CD40L (anti-CD154) turned out to be very efficient in mixed chimerism rodent models (Wekerle et al. 1998). In a molecular chimerism model anti-CD40L was reported to enhance BM engraftment (Bagley et al. 2002c). Anti-CD40L is also effective in preventing sensitization to an allergen (Linhart et al. 2007). Unfortunately, this antibody induces severe thromboembolic side effects in large animals and humans, and is therefore not used in the clinical setting (Kirk et al. 1999; Sidiropoulos and Boumpas 2004). Studies recently published show successful substitution of anti-CD40L by blockade of CD40 in murine models in allo-transplantation (Gilson et al. 2009), but clinical applicability remains uncertain. Blocking alternative co-stimulation pathways may also allow avoidance of anti-CD40L.

HSC engraftment requires—at least some—recipient conditioning. The transplantation of mature T cells instead of HSC in a murine model of molecular chimerism (crossing a MHC I barrier) led to long-lasting central tolerance by re-entry of mature T cells into the thymus (Tian et al. 2004b, 2007b, 2008). Thus, the use of allergen-expressing mature T cells, or other hematopoietic cell populations (McCurry et al. 2006), is an attractive alternative to be explored as a substitute for HSC.

4.2.2 Avoiding Anaphylaxis

Expression of full length allergens on transplanted BM—as in our proof-of-concept studies—implies the risk of anaphylaxis, mostly in the therapeutic but also in the preventive setting. Intracellular expression of an antigen was sufficient to induce T cell tolerance in mice (Tian et al. 2003). Expressing dominant T cell epitopes of allergens on the surface of HSC would conceivably avoid the risk of anaphylaxis, provided that T cell tolerance is sufficient to induce B cell tolerance, as it has been described (Li et al. 2008). Use of small peptides would also facilitate fusion of several dominant T cell epitopes of various allergens to achieve protection toward several allergens at the same time.

5 Conclusion

Preventive and therapeutic tolerance strategies are an important goal for improved medical management of allergies. Cell-based therapies are attractive candidates for development and substantial progress has been achieved in this field at the experimental level. Evaluation of Treg therapy has begun for certain indications and will allow a better appreciation of its usefulness in the treatment of allergy. Molecular chimerism is a powerful experimental approach leading to particularly robust allergen-specific tolerance. Its development is currently at an early proof-of-concept stage, but further progress toward clinical application in the long-term future can be envisioned.

References

Adams AB, Durham MM, Kean L et al (2001) Costimulation blockade, busulfan, and bone marrow promote titratable macrochimerism, induce transplantation tolerance, and correct genetic hemoglobinopathies with minimal myelosuppression. J Immunol 167:1103–1111

Aiuti A, Cattaneo F, Galimberti S et al (2009) Gene therapy for immunodeficiency due to adenosine deaminase deficiency. N Engl J Med 360:447–458

Akdis CA (2006) Allergy and hypersensitivity: mechanisms of allergic disease: autoimmunity/allergy and hypersensitivity. Curr Opin Immunol 18:718–726

Akdis CA, Akdis M (2009) Mechanisms and treatment of allergic disease in the big picture of regulatory T cells. J Allergy Clin Immunol 123:735–746

Akdis M, Verhagen J, Taylor A et al (2004) Immune responses in healthy and allergic individuals are characterized by a fine balance between allergen-specific T regulatory 1 and T helper 2 Cells. J Exp Med 199:1567–1575

Akl A, Jones ND, Rogers N et al (2008) An investigation to assess the potential of CD25highCD4+ T cells to regulate responses to donor alloantigens in clinically stable renal transplant recipients. Transpl Int 21:65–73

Alderuccio F, Murphy K, Toh B-H (2003) Stem cells engineered to express self-antigen to treat autoimmunity. Trend Immunol 24:176–180

Atkinson MA, Leiter EH (1999) The NOD mouse model of type 1 diabetes: as good as it gets? Nat Med 5:601–604

Bagley J, Iacomini J (2003) Gene therapy progress and prospects: gene therapy in organ transplantation. Gene Ther 10:605–611

Bagley J, Wu Y, Sachs DH, Iacomini J (2000) Defining the requirements for peptide recognition in gene therapy-induced T cell tolerance. J Immunol 165:4842–4847

Bagley J, Bracy J, Tian C, Kang E-S, Iacomini J (2002a) Establishing immunological tolerance through the induction of molecular chimerism. Front Biosci 7:1333–1337

Bagley J, Tian C, Sachs DH, Iacomini J (2002b) Induction of T-cell tolerance to an MHC class I alloantigen by gene therapy. Blood 99:4394–4399

Bagley J, Tian C, Sachs DH, Iacomini J (2002c) T cells mediate resistance to genetically modified bone marrow in lethally irradiated recipients. Transplantation 74:1454–1460

Baranyi U, Linhart B, Pilat N et al (2008) Tolerization of a type I allergic immune response through transplantation of genetically modified hematopoietic stem cells. J Immunol 180:8168–8175

Baranyi U, Pilat N, Gattringer M, Wekerle T (2009) A chimerism-based approach to induce tolerance in IgE-mediated allergy. Crit Rev Immunol 29:379–397

Baum C, Dullmann J, Li Z et al (2003) Side effects of retroviral gene transfer into hematopoietic stem cells. Blood 101:2099–2113

Belting M, Wittrup A (2009) Developments in macromolecular drug delivery. Methods Mol Biol 480:1–10

Bigenzahn S, Blaha P, Koporc Z et al (2005) The role of non-deletional tolerance mechanisms in a murine model of mixed chimerism with costimulation blockade. Am J Transplant 5:1237–1247

Billingham RE, Brent L, Medawar PB (1953) "Actively acquired tolerance" of foreign cells. Nature 172:603–606

Blaha P, Bigenzahn S, Koporc Z et al (2003) The influence of immunosuppressive drugs on tolerance induction through bone marrow transplantation with costimulation blockade. Blood 101:2886–2893

Blaha P, Bigenzahn S, Koporc Z, Sykes M, Muehlbacher F, Wekerle T (2005) Short-term immunosuppression facilitates induction of mixed chimerism and tolerance after bone marrow transplantation without cytoreductive conditioning. Transplantation 80:237–243

Bohle B (2008) T cell responses during allergen-specific immunotherapy of Type I allergy. Front Biosci 13:6079–6085

Bracy JL, Iacomini J (2000) Induction of B-cell tolerance by retroviral gene therapy. Blood 96:3008–3015

Bracy J, Iacomini J (2002) Engraftment of genetically modified bone marrow cells in sensitized hosts. Mol Ther 6:252–257

Bracy JL, Sachs DH, Iacomini J (1998) Inhibition of xenoreactive natural antibody production by retroviral gene therapy. Science 281:1845–1847

Bracy JL, Chase CM, Russell PS, Mauiyyedi S, Colvin RB, Iacomini J (2001) Induction of molecular chimerism by gene therapy prevents antibody-mediated heart transplant rejection. Gene Ther 8:1738–1744

Briner TJ, Kuo MC, Keating KM, Rogers BL, Greenstein JL (1993) Peripheral T-cell tolerance in naive and primed mice by subcutaneous injection of peptides from the major cat allergen Fel d I. Proc Natl Acad Sci USA 90(16):7608–7612

Brunstein CG, Miller JS, Cao Q et al (2011) Infusion of ex vivo expanded T regulatory cells in adults transplanted with umbilical cord blood: safety profile and detection kinetics. Blood 117:1061–1070

Bühler LH, Spitzer TR, Sykes M et al (2002) Induction of kidney allograft tolerance after transient lymphohematopoietic chimerism in patients with multiple myeloma and end-stage renal disease. Transplantation 74:1405–1409

Campbell JD, Buckland KF, McMillan SJ et al (2009) Peptide immunotherapy in allergic asthma generates IL-10-dependent immunological tolerance associated with linked epitope suppression. J Exp Med 206:1535–1547

Chai J-G, Xue S, Coe D et al (2005) Regulatory T cells, derived from naive $CD4^{+}CD25^{-}$ T cells by in vitro Foxp3 gene transfer, can induce transplantation tolerance. Transplantation 79:1310–1316

Challacombe SJ, Tomasi TBJR (1980) Systemic tolerance and secretory immunity after oral immunization. J Exp Med 152:1459–1472

Chan J, Ban EJ, Chun KH et al (2008) Transplantation of bone marrow transduced to express self-antigen establishes deletional tolerance and permanently remits autoimmune disease. J Immunol 181:7571–7580

Chatila TA (2005) Role of regulatory T cells in human diseases. J Allergy Clin Immunol 116:949–959

Colson YL, Schuchert MJ, Ildstad ST (2000) The abrogation of allosensitization following the induction of mixed allogeneic chimerism. J Immunol 165:637–644

Copelan EA (2006) Hematopoietic stem-cell transplantation. N Engl J Med 345:1813–1826

Davidson A., Diamond B. (2001) Autoimmune diseases. N Engl J Med 345(5):340–350

Di Ianni M, Falzetti F, Carotti A et al (2011) Tregs prevent GVHD and promote immune reconstitution in HLA-haploidentical transplantation. Blood 117:3921–3928

Down JD, Ploemacher RE (1993) Transient and permanent engraftment potential of murine hematopoietic stem cell subsets: differential effects of host conditioning with gamma radiation and cytotoxic drugs. Exp Hematol 21:913–921

Durham MM, Bingaman AW, Adams AB et al (2000) Administration of anti-CD40 ligand and donor bone marrow leads to hematopoietic chimerism and donor-specific tolerance without cytoreductive conditioning. J Immunol 165:1–4

Eixarch H, Espejo C, Gomez A et al (2009) Tolerance induction in experimental autoimmune encephalomyelitis using non-myeloablative hematopoietic gene therapy with autoantigen. Mol Ther 17:897–905

Emery DW, Shafer GE, Karson EM, Sachs DH, LeGuern C (1993) Retrovirus-mediated transfer and expression of an allogeenic major histocompatibility complex class II DRB cDNA in swine bone marrow cultures. Blood 81:2460–2465

Emery DW, Sablinski T, Shimada H et al (1997) Expression of an allogeneic MHC DRB transgene, through retroviral transduction of bone marrow, induces specific reduction of alloreactivity. Transplantation 64:1414–1423

Faria AMC, Weiner HL (2005) Oral tolerance. Immunol Rev 206:232–259

Fathman CG, Lineberry NB (2007) Molecular mechanisms of CD4+ T-cell anergy. Nat Rev Immunol 7:599–609

Fehr T, Sykes M (2008) Clinical experience with mixed chimerism to induce transplantation tolerance. Transpl Int 21:1118–1135

Feuerer M, Hill JA, Mathis D, Benoist C (2009) Foxp3+ regulatory T cells: differentiation, specification, subphenotypes. Nat Immunol 10:689–695

Fischer-Lougheed JY, Tarantal AF, Shulkin I et al (2006) Gene therapy to inhibit xenoantibody production using lentiviral vectors in non-human primates. Gene Ther 14:49–57
Forman D, Tian C, Iacomini J (2005) Induction of donor-specific tolerance in sublethally irradiated recipients by gene therapy. Mol Ther 12:353–359
Forman D, Kang E-S, Tian C, Paez-Cortez J, Iacomini J (2006) Induction of alloreactive CD4 T cell tolerance in molecular chimeras: a possible role for regulatory T cells. J Immunol 176:3410–3416
Frasca L, Carmichael P, Lechler R, Lombardi G (1997) Anergic T cells effect linked suppression. Eur J Immunol 27:3191–3197
Fraser CC, Sykes M, Lee RS, Sachs DH, LeGuern C (1995) Specific unresponsiveness to a retrovirally-transferred class I antigen is controlled through the helper pathway. J Immunol 154:1587–1595
Friedman A, Weiner HL (1994) Induction of anergy or active suppression following oral tolerance is determined by antigen dosage. Proc Natl Acad Sci USA 91:6688–6692
Fudaba Y, Spitzer TR, Shaffer J et al (2006) Myeloma responses and tolerance following combined kidney and nonmyeloablative marrow transplantation: in vivo and in vitro analyses. Am J Transplant 6:2121–2133
Galili U, Shohet S, Kobrin E, Stults C, Macher B (1988) Man, apes, and Old World monkeys differ from other mammals in the expression of alpha-galactosyl epitopes on nucleated cells. J Biol Chem 263:17755–17762
Gilson CR, Milas Z, Gangappa S et al (2009) Anti-CD40 monoclonal antibody synergizes with CTLA4-Ig in promoting long-term graft survival in murine models of transplantation. J Immunol 183:1625–1635
Hacein-Bey-Abina S, Garrigue A, Wang GP et al (2008) Insertional oncogenesis in 4 patients after retrovirus-mediated gene therapy of SCID-X1. J Clin Invest 118:3132–3142
Hamelmann E, Beyer K, Gruber C et al (2007) Primary prevention of allergy: avoiding risk or providing protection? Clin Exp Allergy 38:233–245
Haselden BM, Kay BA, Larche M (1999) Immunoglobulin E-independent major histocompatibility complex-restricted T cell peptide epitope-induced late asthmatic reactions. J Exp Med 189:1885–1894
Hourinhane JO, Rhodes HL, Jones AM, Veys P, Connett GJ (2005) Resolution of peanut allergy following bone marrow transplantation for primary immunodeficiency. Allergy 60:536–537
Hoyne GF, O'Hehir RE, Wraith DC, Thomas WR, Lamb JR (1993) Inhibition of T cell and antibody responses to house dust mite allergen by inhalation of the dominant T cell epitope in naive and sensitized mice. J Exp Med 178:1783–1788
Hoyne GF, Dallman MJ, Lamb JR (1999) Linked suppression in peripheral T cell tolerance to the house dust mite derived allergen Der p 1. Int Arch Allergy Immunol 118:122–124
Hufnagl K, Winkler B, Focke M et al (2005) Intranasal tolerance induction with polypeptides derived from 3 noncross-reactive major aeroallergens prevents allergic polysensitization in mice. J Allergy Clin Immunol 116:370–376
Hufnagl K, Focke M, Gruber F et al (2008) Airway inflammation induced after allergic polysensitization can be prevented by mucosal but not by systemic administration of polypeptides. Clin Exp Allergy 38:1192–1202
Hutchinson JA, Brem-Exner BG, Riquelme P et al (2008) A cell-based approach to the minimization of immunosuppression in renal transplantation. Transpl Int 21:742–754
Ildstad ST, Sachs DH (1984) Reconstitution with syngeneic plus allogeneic or xenogeneic bone marrow leads to specific acceptance of allografts or xenografts. Nature 307:168–170
Jaeckel E, von Boehmer H, Manns M (2005) Antigen-specific Foxp3 transduced T cells can control established type 1 diabetes. Diabetes 54:306–310
Kang E-S, Iacomini J (2002) Induction of central deletional T cell tolerance by gene therapy. J Immunol 169:1930–1935
Kawai T, Cosimi AB, Spitzer TR et al (2008) HLA-mismatched renal transplantation without maintenance immunosuppression. N Engl J Med 358:353–361

Kearley J, Barker JE, Robinson DS, Lloyd CM (2005) Resolution of airway inflammation and hyperreactivity after in vivo transfer of CD4+CD25+ regulatory T cells is interleukin 10 dependent. J Exp Med 202:1539–1547

Kearley J, Robinson DS, Lloyd CM (2008) CD4+CD25+ regulatory T cells reverse established allergic airway inflammation and prevent airway remodeling. J Allergy Clin Immunol 122:617–624

Kearns-Jonker M, Fischer-Lougheed J, Shulkin I et al (2004) Use of lentiviral vectors to induce long-term tolerance to gal+ heart grafts. Transplantation 77:1748–1754

Khan F, Hallstrand TS, Geddes MN, Henderson WRJ, Storek J (2009) Is allergic disease curable or transferable with allogeneic hematopoietic cell transplantation? Blood 113:279–290

Kirk A, Burkly L, Batty D et al (1999) Treatment with humanized monoclonal antibody against CD154 prevents acute renal allograft rejection in nonhuman primates. Nat Med 5:686–693

Koporc Z, Pilat N, Nierlich P et al (2008) Murine mobilized peripheral blood stem cells have a lower capacity than bone marrow to induce mixed chimerism and tolerance. Am J Transplant 8:2025–2036

Kulig M, Bergmann R, Klette U, Wahn V, Tacke U, Wahn U (1999) Natural course of sensitization to food and inhalant allergens during the first 6 years of life. J Allergy Clin Immunol 103:1173–1179

Larche M, Wraith DC (2005) Peptide-based therapeutic vaccines for allergic and autoimmune diseases. Nat Med 11:S69–S76

Larche M, Akdis CA, Valenta R (2006) Immunological mechanisms of allergen-specific immunotherapy. Nat Rev Immunol 6(10):761–771

Leech MD, Benson RA, deVries A, Fitch PM, Howie SEM (2007) Resolution of Der p1-Induced Allergic Airway Inflammation Is Dependent on CD4+CD25+Foxp3+ regulatory cells. J Immunol 179:7050–7058

LeGuern C (2007) Tolerogenic property of MHC class I and class II molecules: lessons from a gene therapy approach. Front Biosci 12:3133–3139

Levings MK, Sangregorio R, Roncarolo M-R (2001) Human CD25+CD4+ T regulatory cells suppress naive and memory T cell proliferation and can be expanded in vitro without loss of function. J Exp Med 193:1295–1302

Li Y, Ma L, Yin D, Shen J, Chong AS (2008) Long-term control of alloreactive B cell responses by the suppression of T cell help. J Immunol 180:6077–6084

Linhart B, Bigenzahn S, Hartl A et al (2007) Costimulation blockade inhibits allergic sensitization but does not affect established allergy in a murine model of grass pollen allergy. J Immunol 178:3924–3931

LoCascio SA, Morokata T, Chittenden M et al (2010) Mixed chimerism, lymphocyte recovery, and evidence for early donor-specific unresponsiveness in patients receiving combined kidney and bone marrow transplantation to induce tolerance. Transplantation 90:1607–1615

Madsen JC, Superina RA, Wood KJ, Morris PJ (1988) Immunological unresponsiveness induced by recipient cells transfected with donor MHC genes. Nature 332:161–164

Marazuela EG, Rodriguez R, Fernandez-Garcia H, Garcia MS, Villalba M, Batanero E (2008) Intranasal immunization with a dominant T-cell epitope peptide of a major allergen of olive pollen prevents mice from sensitization to the whole allergen. Mol Immunol 45:438–445

Mayfield RS, Hayashi H, Sawada T et al (1997) The mechanism of specific prolongation of class I-mismatched skin grafts induced by retroviral gene therapy. Eur J Immunol 27:1177–1181

McCurry KR, Colvin BL, Zahorchak AF, Thomson AW (2006) Regulatory dendritic cell therapy in organ transplantation. Transpl Int 19:525–538

Meiler F, Zumkehr J, Klunker S, Ruckert B, Akdis CA, Akdis M (2008) In vivo switch to IL-10-secreting T regulatory cells in high dose allergen exposure. J Exp Med 205:2887–2898

Mitsuhashi N, Fischer-Lougheed J, Shulkin I et al (2006) Tolerance induction by lentiviral gene therapy with a nonmyeloablative regimen. Blood 107:2286–2293

Mitsuyasu RT, Merigan TC, Carr A et al (2009) Phase 2 gene therapy trial of an anti-HIV ribozyme in autologous CD34+ cells. Nat Med 15:285–292

Miyara M, Wing K, Sakaguchi S (2009) Therapeutic approaches to allergy and autoimmunity based on FoxP3+ regulatory T-cell activation and expansion. J Allergy Clin Immunol 123:749–755

Nouri-Aria KT, Wachholz PA, Francis JN et al (2004) Grass pollen immunotherapy induces mucosal and peripheral IL-10 responses and blocking IgG activity. J Immunol 172:3252–3259

Ochiai T, Benichou G, Cosimi AB, Kawai T (2007) Induction of allograft tolerance in nonhuman primates and humans. Front Biosci 12:4248–4253

Oldfield WLG, Larché M, Kay AB (2002) Effect of T-cell peptides derived from Fel d 1 on allergic reactions and cytokine production in patients sensitive to cats: a randomised controlled trial. Lancet 360:47–53

Owen RD (1945) Immunogenetic consequences of vascular anastomoses between bovine twins. Science 102:400–401

Peters TR, Bodine DM, McDonagh KT et al (2000) Retrovirus mediated gene transfer of the self antigen MBP into the bone marrow of mice alters resistance to experimental autoimmune encephalomyelitis. J Neuroimmunol 103:51–62

Pilat N, Klaus C, Schwaiger E, Wekerle T (2009) Hurdles to the induction of tolerogenic mixed chimerism. Transplantation 87:S79–S84

Pilat N, Baranyi U, Klaus C et al (2010) Treg-therapy allows mixed chimerism and transplantation tolerance without cytoreductive conditioning. Am J Transplant 10:751–762

Pilat N, Wekerle T (2010) Transplantation tolerance through mixed chimerism. Nat Rev Nephrol 6:594–605

Pree I, Wekerle T (2006) New appproaches to prevent transplant rejection: co-stimulation blockers anti-CD40L and CTLA4Ig. Drug Discov Today: Ther Strateg 3:41–47

Pree I, Pilat N, Wekerle T (2007) Recent progress in tolerance induction through mixed chimerism. Int Arch Allergy Immunol 144:254–266

Qin S, Cobbold SP, Pope H et al (1993) "Infectious" transplantation tolerance. Science 259:974–977

Riley JL, June CH, Blazar BR (2009) Human T regulatory cell therapy: take a billion or so and call me in the morning. Immunity 30:656–665

Roncarolo MG, Battaglia M (2007) Regulatory T-cell immunotherapy for tolerance to self antigens and alloantigens in humans. Nat Rev Immunol 7:585–598

Roncarolo MG, Gregori S, Battaglia M, Bacchetta R, Fleischhauer K, Levings MK (2006) Interleukin-10-secreting type 1 regulatory T cells in rodents and humans. Immunol Rev 212:28–50

Sakaguchi S (2005) Naturally arising Foxp3-expressing CD25+CD4+ regulatory T cells in immunologic tolerance to self and non-self. Nat Immunol 6:345–352

Sakaguchi S, Powrie F (2007) Emerging challenges in regulatory T cell function and biology. Science 317:627–629

Sakaguchi S, Yamaguchi T, Nomura T, Ono M (2008) Regulatory T cells and immune tolerance. Cell 133:775–787

Schiopu A, Wood KJ (2008) Regulatory T cells: hypes and limitations. Curr Opin Organ Transplant 13:333–338

Shafer GE, Emery DW, Gustafsson K et al (1991) Expression of a swine class II gene in murine bone marrow hematopoietic cells by retroviral-mediated gene transfer. Proc Natl Acad Sci USA 88:9760–9764

Sidiropoulos PI, Boumpas DT (2004) Lessons learned from anti-CD40L treatment in systemic lupus erythematosus patients. Lupus 13:391–397

Singer A, Hathcock KS, Hodes RJ (1981) Self recognition in allogeneic radiation chimeras. A radiation resistant host element dictates the self specificity and immune response gene phenotype of T-helper cells. J Exp Med 153:1286–1301

Snanoudj R, de Preneuf H, Creput C et al (2006) Costimulation blockade and its possible future use in clinical transplantation. Transpl Int 19:693–704

Sonntag KC, Emery DW, Yasumoto A et al (2001) Tolerance to solid organ transplants through transfer of MHC class II genes. J Clin Invest 107:65–71

Storek J, Vliagoftis H, Grizel A et al (2011) Allergy transfer with hematopoietic cell transplantation from an unrelated donor. Bone Marrow Transplant 46:605–606
Sykes M (2001) Mixed chimerism and transplant tolerance. Immunity 14:417–424
Sykes M, Sheard MA, Sachs DH (1988) Graft-versus-host-related immunosuppression is induced in mixed chimeras by alloresponses against either host or donor lymphohematopoietic cells. J Exp Med 168:2391–2396
Sykes M, Ohdan H, Manilay JO, Wekerle T, Yang YG (1998) Hematopoietic chimerism and tolerance of T cells, B cells, and NK cells. Transpl Proc 30:420
Takeuchi Y, Ito H, Kurtz J, Wekerle T, Ho L, Sykes M (2004) Earlier low-dose TBI or DST overcomes $CD8^{+}$ T-cell-mediated alloresistance to allogeneic marrow in recipients of anti-CD40L. Am J Transplant 4:31–40
Thomas CE, Ehrhardt A, Kay MA (2003) Progress and problems with the use of viral vectors for gene therapy. Nature Rev Genet 4:346–358
Tian C, Bagley J, Kaye J, Iacomini J (2003) Induction of T cell tolerance to a protein expressed in the cytoplasm through retroviral-mediated gene transfer. J Gene Med 5:359–365
Tian C, Bagley J, Cretin N, Seth N, Wucherpfennig KW, Iacomini J (2004a) Prevention of type 1 diabetes by gene therapy. J Clin Invest 114:969–978
Tian C, Bagley J, Forman D, Iacomini J (2004b) Induction of central tolerance by mature T cells. J Immunol 173:7217–7222
Tian C, Bagley J, Iacomini J (2006) Persistence of antigen is required to maintain transplantation tolerance induced by genetic modification of bone marrow stem cells. Am J Transplant 6:2202–2207
Tian C, Ansari MJI, Paez-Cortez J et al (2007a) Induction of robust diabetes resistance and prevention of recurrent type 1 diabetes following islet transplantation by gene therapy. J Immunol 179:6762–6769
Tian C, Bagley J, Iacomini J (2007b) Homeostatic expansion permits T Cells to re-enter the thymus and deliver antigen in a tolerogenic fashion. Am J Transplant 7:1934–1941
Tian C, Yuan X, Bagley J, Blazar BR, Sayegh MH, Iacomini J (2008) Induction of transplantation tolerance by combining non-myeloablative conditioning with delivery of alloantigen by T cells. Clin Immunol 127:130–137
Trzonkowski P, Bieniaszewska M, Juscinska J et al (2009) First-in-man clinical results of the treatment of patients with graft versus host disease with human ex vivo expanded CD4+CD25+CD127-Tregulatory cells. Clin Immunol 133:22–26
Valenta R (2002) The future of antigen-specific immunotherapy of allergy. Nat Rev Immunol 2:446–453
Valenta R, Kraft D (2002) From allergen structure to new forms of allergen-specific immunotherapy. Curr Opin Immunol 14:718–727
VandenDriessche T, Ivics Z, Izsvak Z, Chuah MKL (2009) Emerging potential of transposons for gene therapy and generation of induced pluripotent stem cells. Blood 114:1461–1468
Vercelli D (2008) Discovering susceptibility genes for asthma and allergy. Nat Rev Immunol 8:169–182
von Boehmer H, Kisielow P (2006) Negative selection of the T-cell repertoire: where and when does it occur? Immunol Rev 209:284–289
Vrtala S, Sperr W, Reimitzer I et al (1993) cDNA cloning of a major allergen from timothy grass (*Phleum pratense*) pollen; characterization of the recombinant Phl pV allergen. J Immunol 151:4773–4781
Wachholz PA, Durham SR (2003) Induction of 'blocking' IgG antibodies during immunotherapy. Clin Exp Allergy 33:1171–1174
Webb SR, Morris C, Sprent J (1990) Extrathymic tolerance of mature T cells: clonal elimination as a consequence of immunity. Cell 63:1249–1256
Wekerle T, Sykes M (2001) Mixed chimerism and transplantation tolerance. Annu Rev Med 52:353–370

Wekerle T, Sayegh MH, Hill J et al (1998) Extrathymic T cell deletion and allogeneic stem cell engraftment induced with costimulatory blockade is followed by central T cell tolerance. J Exp Med 187:2037–2044

Wekerle T, Kurtz J, Ito H et al (2000) Allogeneic bone marrow transplantation with co-stimulatory blockade induces macrochimerism and tolerance without cytoreductive host treatment. Nature Med 6:464–469

Wekerle T, Kurtz J, Bigenzahn S, Takeuchi Y, Sykes M (2002) Mechanisms of transplant tolerance induction using costimulatory blockade. Curr Opin Immunol 14:592–600

Wekerle T, Blaha P, Koporc Z, Bigenzahn S, Pusch M, Muehlbacher F (2003) Mechanisms of tolerance induction through the transplantation of donor hematopoietic stem cells: central versus peripheral. Transplantation 75:21S–25S

Wells HG (1911) Studies on the chemistry of anaphylaxis. III. Experiments with isolated proteins, especially those of the hens egg. J Infect Dis 9:147–171

Wild C, Wallner M, Hufnagl K et al (2007) A recombinant allergen chimer as novel mucosal vaccine candidate for prevention of multi-sensitivities. Allergy 62:33–41

Winkler B, Hufnagl K, Spittler A et al (2006) The role of Foxp3+ T cells in long-term efficacy of prophylactic and therapeutic mucosal tolerance induction in mice. Allergy 61:173–180

Xu B, Scott DW (2004) A novel retroviral gene therapy approach to inhibit specific antibody production and suppress experimental autoimmune encephalomyelitis induced by MOG and MBP. Clin Immunol 111:47–52

Xu B, Haviernik P, Wolfraim LA, Bunting KD, Scott DW (2006) Bone marrow transplantation combined with gene therapy to induce antigen-specific tolerance and ameliorate EAE. Mol Ther 13:42–48

Yang J, Brook MO, Carvalho-Gaspar M et al (2007) Allograft rejection mediated by memory T cells is resistant to regulation. Proc Natl Acad Sci USA 104:19954–19959

Yolcu ES, Askenasy N, Singh NP, Cherradi S-EL, Shirwan H (2002) Cell membrane modification for rapid display of proteins as a novel means of immunomodulation: FasL-decorated cells prevent islet graft rejection. Immunity 17:795–808

Zamvil SS, Steinman L (1990) The T lymphocyte in experimental allergic encephalomyelitis. Annu Rev Immunol 8:579–621

Index

Current Topics in Microbiology and Immunology (2011) 352: 181–182
DOI: 10.1007/978-3-642-20054-0